Acting Edition

Last Night and the Night Before

by Donnetta Lavinia Grays

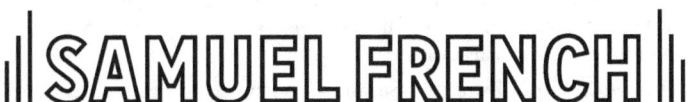

Copyright © 2024 by Donnetta Lavinia Grays
All Rights Reserved

LAST NIGHT AND THE NIGHT BEFORE is fully protected under the copyright laws of the United States of America, the British Commonwealth, including Canada, and all member countries of the Berne Convention for the Protection of Literary and Artistic Works, the Universal Copyright Convention, and/or the World Trade Organization conforming to the Agreement on Trade Related Aspects of Intellectual Property Rights. All rights, including professional and amateur stage productions, recitation, lecturing, public reading, motion picture, radio broadcasting, television, online/digital production, and the rights of translation into foreign languages are strictly reserved.

ISBN 978-0-573-71106-0

www.concordtheatricals.com
www.concordtheatricals.co.uk

FOR PRODUCTION INQUIRIES

UNITED STATES AND CANADA
info@concordtheatricals.com
1-866-979-0447

UNITED KINGDOM AND EUROPE
licensing@concordtheatricals.co.uk
020-7054-7298

Each title is subject to availability from Concord Theatricals Corp., depending upon country of performance. Please be aware that *LAST NIGHT AND THE NIGHT BEFORE* may not be licensed by Concord Theatricals Corp. in your territory. Professional and amateur producers should contact the nearest Concord Theatricals Corp. office or licensing partner to verify availability.

CAUTION: Professional and amateur producers are hereby warned that *LAST NIGHT AND THE NIGHT BEFORE* is subject to a licensing fee. The purchase, renting, lending or use of this book does not constitute a license to perform this title(s), which license must be obtained from Concord Theatricals Corp. prior to any performance. Performance of this title(s) without a license is a violation of federal law and may subject the producer and/or presenter of such performances to civil penalties. Both amateurs and professionals considering a production are strongly advised to apply to the appropriate agent before starting rehearsals, advertising, or booking a theatre. A licensing fee must be paid whether the title(s) is presented for charity or gain and whether or not admission is charged. Professional/Stock licensing fees are quoted upon application to Concord Theatricals Corp.

This work is published by Samuel French, an imprint of Concord Theatricals Corp.

No one shall make any changes in this title(s) for the purpose of production. No part of this book may be reproduced, stored in a retrieval system, scanned, uploaded, or transmitted in any form, by any means, now known or yet to be invented, including mechanical, electronic, digital, photocopying, recording, videotaping, or otherwise, without the prior written permission of the publisher. No one shall share this title(s), or any part of this title(s), through any social media or file hosting websites.

For all inquiries regarding motion picture, television, online/digital and other media rights, please contact Concord Theatricals Corp.

MUSIC AND THIRD-PARTY MATERIALS USE NOTE

Licensees are solely responsible for obtaining formal written permission from copyright owners to use copyrighted music and/or other copyrighted third-party materials (e.g. artworks, logos) in the performance of this play and are strongly cautioned to do so. If no such permission is obtained by the licensee, then the licensee must use only original music and materials that the licensee owns and controls. Licensees are solely responsible and liable for clearances of all third-party copyrighted materials, including without limitation music, and shall indemnify the copyright owners of the play(s) and their licensing agent, Concord Theatricals Corp., against any costs, expenses, losses and liabilities arising from the use of such copyrighted third-party materials by licensees. For music, please contact the appropriate music licensing authority in your territory for the rights to any incidental music.

IMPORTANT BILLING AND CREDIT REQUIREMENTS

If you have obtained performance rights to this title, please refer to your licensing agreement for important billing and credit requirements.

LAST NIGHT AND THE NIGHT BEFORE received its world premiere at the Denver Center for the Performing Arts on January 25, 2019. The performance was directed by Valerie Curtis-Newton, with scenic design by Matthew Smucker, costume design by Melanie Burgess, lighting design by Mary Louise Geiger, sound design by Larry D. Fowler Jr., voice and dialect coaching by Dwight Bacquie, dramaturgy by Jacqueline E. Lawton, and casting by Harriet Bass, CSA and Grady Soapes, CSA. The production stage manager was Randall K. Lum, the assistant stage manager was Kristen O'Connor, and the apprentice stage manager was Wayne Breyer. The cast was as follows:

SAM . . . . Zaria Kelley
MONIQUE . . . . Keona Welch
REGGIE . . . . Sharod Choyce
RACHEL . . . . Bianca Laverne Jones
NADIMA . . . . Erin Cherry

LAST NIGHT AND THE NIGHT BEFORE made its Chicago premiere at Steppenwolf Theater Company on April 16, 2023. The performance was directed by Valerie Curtis-Newton, with scenic design by Regina Garcia, costume design by Izumi Inaba, lighting design by Mary Louise Geiger, sound design by Larry D. Fowler Jr., voice and dialect coaching by Gigi Buffington, intimacy choreography by Kristen Baity, and casting by JC Clementz. The producing director was Tom Pearl, the production stage manager was Laura D. Glenn, the assistant stage manager was Jaclynn Joslin, and the assistant director was Alex Dauphin. The cast was as follows:

SAM . . . . Kaylah Renee Jones
MONIQUE . . . . Ayanna Bria Bakari
REGGIE . . . . Namir Smallwood
RACHEL . . . . Sydney Charles
NADIMA . . . . Jessica Dean Turner

Aliyana Nicole rotated the role of Sam with Ms. Jones after opening night.

DEVELOPMENT HISTORY

LAST NIGHT AND THE NIGHT BEFORE (formerly *SAM*) was developed in New York City partly through Naked Angels' Tuesdays@9 open reading series (Andrea Cirie and Joe Danisi, Creative Directors) and was given a more formal public reading with Naked Angels (Andy Donald, Artistic Director) on March 4, 2013, in their 1st Mondays reading series. The reading was directed by Colette Robert.

Excerpts of the play were read as part of Classical Theatre of Harlem's Playwrights Playground on March 11, 2013. The play was featured as part of Classical Theatre of Harlem's Future Classics Reading Series (Ty Jones, Artistic Director; Shawn Rene Graham, Curator) on December 16, 2013. Colette Robert directed.

In November 2014 the play was given a reading through The Actors Studio's Playwright/Directors Unit of which Donnetta was a member. Woodie King Jr. directed.

The play received an extensive workshop May 4–9, 2015, through Portland Stage Company's Little Festival of the Unexpected (Anita Stewart, Artistic Director). Sally Wood directed.

The play received an extensive rehearsal and reading November 3–9, 2015, as part of Orlando Shakespeare Theater's Annual PlayFest (Jim Helsinger, Artistic Director; Cynthia White, Curator). Lisa Wolpe directed.

The play received a reading as part of LAByrinth Theater Company's Barn Series (Mimi O'Donnell, Artistic Director; Kevin Snipes, Artistic Associate/Curator) on June 10, 2016. Colette Robert directed.

The play received further development as part of Denver Center for the Arts' (Kent Thompson, Artistic Director; Douglas Langworthy, Director of New Play Development) Colorado New Play Summit, February 14–26, 2017. Valerie Curtis-Newton directed. Lauren Whitehead was dramaturg.

CHARACTERS

SAM – A ten-year-old girl. Smart. Sharp. Inquisitive. Dark. Loving.

MONIQUE – Sam's mother. Early–mid twenties. A poet. A lost soul. Loving.

REGGIE – Sam's father. Early–mid twenties. Loving to a fault. Boyish. Unfaltering.

RACHEL – Sam's aunt. Monique's sister. Mid thirties. Warm-hearted. Steely but with cracks. Guilt-ridden. Loving.

NADIMA – Rachel's girlfriend. Mid thirties. Playful. Charming. Funny. Fiercely protective. Loving.

SETTING & TIME

The play takes place today in a smartly – yet not overly – decorated brownstone in Brooklyn, just outside that brownstone, back in time a few moments to "Vixten," Georgia, and presently on an unnamed city street.

There should be a way for the interior and exterior of the brownstone to be simultaneously visible. The kitchen should be somewhat visible from the living room and should assume that a sit-in kitchen table is hidden.

Vixten, Georgia, should not live in the concrete world. Along with the unnamed street, Vixten should either drape around or flow into the Brooklyn spaces as they are conjured. Georgia red clay should feature prominently into the design and may bleed into the Brooklyn space.

Each scene should flow into the next holding the lyricism of the play at the forefront. An air of what has just happened should stay inside of what is happening now. Past and present are liquid. Limit the use of blackouts.

AUTHOR'S NOTES

Sam is in no way a "magical" child. The hand games she plays or is introduced to should inform the development of each flashback and give us insight into her mental state. Each song has a specific meaning as it relates to those scenes and serves as an active conjuring or wishful reinventing of her circumstances. Monique holds the power of this imagination as well.

Rachel and Nadima are lesbians. Simply and affirmatively. They exist in both feminine and masculine space fluidly. Resist any impulse to emulate a heteronormative relationship or define them through a heteronormative gaze. Allow their love to be complex and for their story to be rooted in that complex love.

Resist the urge to paint Nadima with the singular brush of brashness. Her lightness and humor, balanced with her sense of protection for Rachel, are crucial to understanding their love story.

Monique, Reggie, and Sam have a secret. The careful calibration of what is true in what they reveal to Rachel and Nadima will determine if the audience gets ahead of it or not. Aim for subtlety. Allow Sam to come into Rachel emotionally and Rachel room to struggle in her adopted role as caretaker/adoptive mother.

The Vixten dialect is one that I imagine with soft notes of Gullah Geechee sounds that one might find in the city decedents of Coastal Georgia/South Carolina Lowcountry people (Think: The rapper T.I. and his wife Tiny).

We get a soft Gullah Geechee line from Rachel in Act Two, Scene One:

"Girl! You ain't only gonna be actin' 'umanish you gwine be an actualized 'uman!"

Which translates to: "You ain't only going to be acting 'woman-ish' you are going to be an actualized woman!"

Slashes (/) indicate overlapping. Dashes (–) indicate cut-offs or a quick turn of thought.

Brackets ([]) indicate subtext.

Finally, Monique has several quick changes. More than one dresser and/or underdressing will be needed. Apologies from the playwright.

ACT ONE

Prologue

(A moonlit night. It is quiet. Then, the gently increasing sounds of a shovel piercing the earth and the work [the breath, grunts, and aches] of a man digging that earth fill the space. The digging is purposeful, intense, and almost coming to an end. Lights partially reveal a **YOUNG MAN** *in motion – sweat on his brow, determined. He wears a white work shirt, dark pants, rubber gloves, and dustcovers on his shoes. Maybe even a hair net. Blood and dirt have made a mess of his clothes. He adjusts a gun in his waistband. At his feet is a body wrapped in a blanket and tied tightly around the ankles, at the waist, and at the shoulders with tape or rope or whatever he could find. Exhausted, the* **MAN** *gulps water from a bottle as though he has never tasted such relief. Then, the sound of a swelling distant breath fills the air. It is panicked. Short. Fearful. Just over the* **MAN**'s *shoulder lights partially reveal a* **YOUNG GIRL** *sitting knees to chest. Her eyes transfixed on the body. She is a little done up. Almost as if she's headed for Sunday school. A contrary figure in such a dark place. The* **MAN**, *sensing a presence, turns but sees no one. He returns to the hole he has dug. Studies it. He is tired*

but there is more work to be done. He drags the body as far as he can and kicks it into the freshly made grave. He spits into the grave. Wipes his brow. Turns back to check his surroundings. Sees no one. A fresh panicked breath fights with the words stuck in the little girl's throat as she tries to mouth some sweet inaudible thing. Lights begin to fade on the **GRAVEDIGGER** *and the gently decreasing sounds of a shovel and the work [the breath, grunts, and aches] of a man returning the earth from which it came. Just as lights begin to rise on a* **YOUNG GIRL** *meeting a Brooklyn morning and the increasing sound of her nearly stunted voice...)*

SAM.
Miss Mary Mack Mack Mack
All dressed in black black black
With silvah buttons buttons buttons
All down her back back back

Scene One

(The early morning light fully reveals **SAM** *[ten] as she sits knees to chest curbside on a brown-stoned tree-lined Brooklyn street. Sounds of African, Caribbean, and hip-hop music meld with Islamic and Jewish prayers and the sounds of traffic. She continues to nervously sing/play this hand game by herself.)*

SAM.

She asked her mother mother mother

For fifteen cents...cents...

(A car zooms by playing some loud calypso song. It startles her a bit. She covers her ears. Breathes deeply. Tries a different song. Whispers to herself as she lightly goes through the motions.)

Let's get the rhythm of head *(Nods head.)*

Let's get the rhythm of the hands *(Clap, Clap.)*

Let's get the rhythm of feet *(Stomp, Stomp.)*

Let's get the rhythm...

(She is lost in her anxiety and the song trails off. She holds her knees closer to her chest.)

*(***MONIQUE***, Sam's mom, enters agitated looking at a piece of paper. She is in her early twenties and could pass for Sam's sister. She wears jeans, t-shirt, sneakers, and hoodie. She stops in front of* **SAM** *who stares at her mother like a stranger. Or maybe even a ghost. There is a held tension between these two.)*

It's right here.

MONIQUE. Why you ain't said nothin'?

SAM. I did, mama. You ain't *listen* to me!

MONIQUE. Watch ya mouth.

SAM. Yes ma'am.

MONIQUE. Fix ya'self up.

> (**MONIQUE** *pats* **SAM**'s *hair back with her hands.*)

Lemme see ya teeth! Come on. Warm the sun up, baby.

> (**SAM** *forces a smile.*)

There you go. Nah, you gonna smile jus' like that when we see ya aunties, 'kay?

SAM. Yes ma'am.

MONIQUE. Gotta to put on a good show fah they bougie asses.

SAM. Yes ma'am.

MONIQUE. Nah don't go repeatin' that alright.

SAM. *(Gets anxious. Starts to lose her breath.)* Yes ma'–

MONIQUE. *(Taking* **SAM** *by the shoulders.)* Unh uh, now. Come on. Look at me. Look at mama, baby. Breathe. Breathe fah me.

> *(They breathe together and after a moment* **SAM** *calms down.)*

Better?

SAM. *(Uncertain.)* Yes ma'am.

MONIQUE. Yeah. You good. You gonna be jus' fine. 'Kay?

> *(She kisses her daughter's forehead.* **SAM** *recoils a little.* **MONIQUE** *registers this.)*

Sho you ain't hungry?

SAM. *(Whiney. Exhausted.)* Mama, I *said* I wasn't –.

MONIQUE. *(Sucks teeth.)* Hush up! No. You 'bout to *eat* inna minute.

> *(***SAM*** pouts. They climb the stairs of the brownstone.* ***MONIQUE*** *rings the bell. Then, knocks loudly at the door. They wait. She knocks again.)*

SAM. Maybe they ain't home.

MONIQUE. *(Snaps.)* Dammit I said hush!

> *(***MONIQUE*** *looks at* ***SAM*** *with a little desperation. She knocks again. Then, the sounds of* ***WOMEN*** *laughing as the lights rise on the inside of the brownstone. Another knock. After a moment, an attractive woman in her mid thirties –* ***NADIMA*** *– appears in the bedroom doorway adjusting her robe.)*

RACHEL. *(From the bedroom. Pouty.)* Get rid of them and come back!

NADIMA. *(Flirty. To the bedroom.)* Woman, if you move a single solitary inch... my god.

> *(***SAM*** *stands behind her mother shyly.* ***MONIQUE*** *rings the doorbell.* ***NADIMA*** *turns on a light to the living room heading toward the accosted front door.)*

RACHEL. *(From the bedroom.)* Tell them our souls are saved and we *have* heard the good news!

> *(They laugh.)*

NADIMA. Ha! *(To the door.)* Please do not knock my door down!

*(**NADIMA** looks through the eyehole. Stops. Looks through the eyehole again. Hesitates. Opens the door. An awkward silence as the **WOMEN** stand not quite knowing what to say.)*

MONIQUE. *(Big and playfully.)* Hey!

NADIMA. *(Beat. In shock, she calls back toward the bedroom.)* Babe...? It's for you!

*(**RACHEL** – mid thirties and warm-hearted – calls sleepily from the bedroom.)*

RACHEL. You can't handle it?

NADIMA. It's a...a surprise.

*(**NADIMA** crosses into the bedroom leaving **MONIQUE** to hang back waiting uncomfortably. **RACHEL** enters from the bedroom adjusting her robe.)*

RACHEL. *(Seeing **MONIQUE**. Her stomach sinks.)* Jesus...

MONIQUE. Recognize the face?

RACHEL. Neekie. Neekie?! Oh, my god! What are you [doing] –

MONIQUE. Sammie, get from behind me 'n say hey tah ya auntie.

RACHEL. Sam? Oh, my god, Sam!

SAM. Hey, Aunt Rachel.

MONIQUE. She big right?

RACHEL. I was just about to say. Let me look at you.

*(**SAM** goes to her aunt.)*

Lord have mercy... *(Calls to the bedroom.)* Baby, Sam with her!

(**NADIMA** *reappears from the bedroom now dressed in pajamas.*)

NADIMA. Sam? I didn't see the kid. / Hey, munchkin.

RACHEL. I know, right?

SAM. Hey Aunt / Dima

RACHEL. You are so big. Look at your hair –

NADIMA. I didn't see you / standing back there.

MONIQUE. Hidin' behind me. / Tryna act shy.

RACHEL. Who did that for you? Your mama?

SAM. Yes ma'am.

(Silence.)

RACHEL. Well, don't just stand there. Why y'all just standing there?

MONIQUE. Well, let us in, girl!

RACHEL. *(Ushering them in.)* Oh shoot. Right! Look at me. Come on in! Y'all come on in here.

NADIMA. Uh… Coffee?

RACHEL. You want some coffee?

MONIQUE. Yeah that'd be good.

(**NADIMA** *exits to the kitchen.*)

(To **RACHEL.***)* Also, Sam a lil hungry if y'all got anythang.

(**MONIQUE** *cuts a look to* **SAM** *who cuts a look right back. They are still quietly fighting.*)

RACHEL. Nadima, –

NADIMA. I heard.

(Beat.)

RACHEL. Wow!

MONIQUE. Yeah.

>   *(An uneasy beat.)*

RACHEL. You're here.

MONIQUE. *(Jokingly.)* Well, you know, we was drivin' around n'...we was jus' in the neighborhood.

RACHEL. From Georgia?

MONIQUE. So...

>   *(Beat.)*

RACHEL. *(Calling to the kitchen.)* Nadima, Sam's coming in the kitchen to help you out! *(To* **SAM.***)* Sam, go on in there and let Aunt Dima know what you want to eat, baby.

SAM. Yes ma'am.

>   *(They watch her reluctantly exit.* **MONIQUE** *a little satisfied.)*

RACHEL. Where's Reggie?

MONIQUE. He ain't in the car.

>   *(Beat.)*

RACHEL. Why don't you have a seat, baby.

MONIQUE. I been on my ass fah over ten hours, girl. Feels good bein' on my feet.

RACHEL. You got uh, bags...or anything?

MONIQUE. Little bit 'a stuff out in the car. My car gonna be alright out 'dey?

RACHEL. Should be.

>   *(Beat.)*

Please start talking.

MONIQUE. *(Laughs nervously.)* Girl... *(Looks up.)* Gre'd day! How far up this ceilin' go? This is nice.

RACHEL. Thank you.

MONIQUE. I like this block too. But, I can live wit'out all that traffic I can tell ya that right nah! Thank I lost 'bout ten years offa my life. The noise is like...ugh!! Forever wit' all that honkin'!

RACHEL. You get used to it.

MONIQUE. You move here what? 'Bout two – three years / ago?

RACHEL. Two. Neekie?

MONIQUE. He gone. Yep yep yep. Far from Vixten by now I 'magine.

RACHEL. Where?

MONIQUE. I don't know. A man is a...complicated mess of a thang, ain't they? Well, hell you don't know.

RACHEL. Monique.

MONIQUE. No, ...I ain't tryna be funny. I'm jus' tryna fix my head 'round a couple thangs. An' it's complicated. It's all a lil messed up right nah.

(Beat.)

He uh lost his job. Chil' they downsized that plant so much it ain't even 'nere no more hardly.

RACHEL. Carson's shutting down?

MONIQUE. Jus' bout. D'ere's a big ole hole in town. *You* wouldn't recognize it anymore that's fah sure. *(Off* **RACHEL.***)* Anyway...he tried gettin' other work. He even applied tah a couple 'a fast food places. Like wit' me? But he ain't wanna do that really. His pride get in the way... An' he was on unemployment fah a minute. Then that ran out 'n –

RACHEL. And so did *he*?

MONIQUE. That's the story.

RACHEL. Short story.

MONIQUE. Well, that's how it is.

RACHEL. *(Carefully.)* Monique, did he hurt you? / Did he put his hands –

MONIQUE. Oh no! No! That ain't – No. God no. You know Reggie. He a good man.

RACHEL. Is he?

MONIQUE. You *know* he is! He just don't... He *real* good, Rach. I mean, I seen that man do...extraordinary thangs over his whole life.

RACHEL. His *whole life*? Neekie, he's twenty-six years old! Ain't no *whole* yet.

MONIQUE. He just like tah be big. You know *man-ish* 'n all that shit.

> (**SAM** *bursts from the kitchen. She has wrapped up whatever food she was given and folded it into her dress to carry.* **NADIMA** *trails her eating an English muffin Monique's coffee in hand.*)

SAM. *(Still hot.)* I could eat outside? *(Checks her attitude. Studies her feet.)* Aunt Dima said to ask if I could eat outside onna stairs.

> (**MONIQUE**, *knowing she's lost this battle, stares at* **SAM**.)

RACHEL. Um...sure, baby. If that's alright with –

SAM. *(Head down.)* I just wanna...see stuff.

MONIQUE. *(Reaching down to touch* **SAM**'s *face.)* You stay right out dey on them steps where we can see ya.

> (**SAM** *doesn't return* **MONIQUE***'s gaze. Pulls away sharply.* **RACHEL** *and* **NADIMA** *clock the tension.* **NADIMA** *opens the door for* **SAM** *to exit. Glances at her from the window. Hands* **MONIQUE** *her coffee.*)

What you gave her?

NADIMA. She didn't want much. Cheese and crackers.

MONIQUE. Well...dat's her. Picky eater.

NADIMA. Hm. Trip that long with a picky eater?

MONIQUE. *(Narrowing her eyes.)* I *feeds* my child, Nadima.

NADIMA. I didn't say / you don't.

MONIQUE. Stopped 'n got her somethin' fo' we left *and* in Tennessee so –

RACHEL. Whoa whoa whoa. Tennessee?

NADIMA. The hell kinda route did you take?!

RACHEL. *(Incredulous.)* The *long* way.

MONIQUE. That's the long way?

RACHEL. Girl!

MONIQUE. Musta got bad directions.

NADIMA. You could have just gone online –

MONIQUE. Well, maybe some people ain't got no computer. You ever thought about that? I went old school. Rand McNally okay.

NADIMA. Fine. Fine.

> (*She sips her coffee. Bites her muffin.*)

So, what's the deal?

RACHEL. We were just / getting to that.

MONIQUE. I know. I know. I jus' come up here 'n –. Oh, man! Y'all gotta be tah work?

NADIMA. That's the usual / chain of events.

RACHEL. I can cancel my class –

MONIQUE. *(Apologetically.)* Aw naw. I jus' bus' up y'alls / situation.

NADIMA. I can't hang around too much longer. Inspector's coming to see the property.

MONIQUE. Y'all, I'm sorry. / I shouldna come bustin' in...

RACHEL. Just. Relax okay. Nadima, don't you need to get ready?

NADIMA. Yep. *(Takes a quick bite of her English muffin.)* So?

MONIQUE. What?

NADIMA. Are you uh, just here for the day? Dropping by to say hello?

RACHEL. *(Grins. Shakes her head.)* Nadima.

NADIMA. Have you reserved a room at the Marriott for the evening?

RACHEL. Stop it, / baby.

MONIQUE. I'm tired, okay. I been on the road all night. You could at least *act* like you happy tah see me.

NADIMA. See, I'm not quite sure if I am just yet.

RACHEL. Nadima!

MONIQUE. Huh! Thanks for the coffee.

RACHEL. Nadima, go shit 'n shower please. I'm gonna sit here and listen to what my little sister has to say.

MONIQUE. Yeah, I'm tryna have a private conversation / wit' my sister!

NADIMA. A private conversation? In my house?

MONIQUE. Oh, you the only one stay here?

RACHEL. Honey, please you're / gonna have to –

MONIQUE. You picked a *choice* one / sis, ya hear me!

NADIMA. Disrespect me one more / time –

RACHEL. Okay, ladies that's enough! You've said your hellos. Now, Sam is out there. I'm sure she can hear just about everything. And we don't need Mrs. Anderson coming down talking about her "concerns." So please.

> *(The ladies cease fire.)*

NADIMA. Okay. Okay. Come here.

> *(She takes **RACHEL** aside. Holds her around the waist with one arm. Looks her in the eye.)*

Take care of this.

> *(Presses her hand on **RACHEL**'s heart.)*

Take care of this.

> *(Presses her hand on **RACHEL**'s head. Kisses it.)*

RACHEL. I will.

> *(**RACHEL** taps her fingers to her own lips.)*

Take care of *this*.

NADIMA. With pleasure.

> *(They kiss. They smile. A bit of their lovers' routine.)*

Good morning. I'll be right in there if you need me. Love you.

RACHEL. Love you too.

(**NADIMA** *exits to the bedroom.*)

RACHEL. *(To* **MONIQUE**.*)* I'm sorry about –

MONIQUE. Don't apologize fah her! That chick is outta her goddamn min'. Seriously, *that's* the one ya end up wit', hunh?

RACHEL. Watch it alright.

MONIQUE. Lord knows why you want to be with a woman in the first place. / That right they is some –

RACHEL. Reggie lost his job…

MONIQUE. Hunh? Right! He was tryna find work –

RACHEL. And he left you and the kid.

(**MONIQUE** *nods.*)

What *are* you gonna do?

MONIQUE. Hunh?

RACHEL. To be clear; I was apologizing not for *what* my girlfriend said but for *how* she said it. She's justified.

(Beat.)

Now, Neekie, I have had your back on some deep-ass shit. Some *crazy*-ass shit. Okay? And I wake up today and you got *Sam* up here with you. Half a story in your hand. You have to give me *something*.

(*Beat.* **MONIQUE** *starts to cry.* **RACHEL** *embraces her sister.*)

MONIQUE. I done messed up… I been messin' up fah a minute, ya know. An' it cost me. It come tah a head.

(**MONIQUE** *releases from the hug. She walks around the room. Collecting her stories from the walls it seems.*)

I jus'... I jus' figured he needed a lil breathin' room tah clear his head 'a somethin'. Dealin' wit' so much bein' laid-off 'n everythang. He'd been hangin' out at The Blue Room. And I'm sittin' home. Phone ain't ringin'. But then it was a night, then a day, a week 'n I still ain't heard from 'im.

RACHEL. He went out one night and never came back? You call the cops? Ask his friends?

MONIQUE. Ain't no cops in southern Georgia concerned about a missin' nigga now come on. Ain't nobody see'd nor heard from 'im. 'Course I asked around. People shut they door in my face. I'm *that* woman, ya know. Embarrasin'. I don't know...

> *(As she paces she happens upon a small picture in her pocket. Turns it over. Examines it. Shifts.)*

...then I found *this* in his...in his pants pocket.

> *(Handing over a picture of an attractive woman.)*

RACHEL. No, Reggie, no...

MONIQUE. D'ere's a uh number on the back.

RACHEL. You called it?

MONIQUE. I jus' listened to her sayin' "hello" over 'n over again. Keeping time to her breath. Like it was damn near makin' a song. He left wit' what he had on his back 'n nothin' else...to be wit' her. That's his daughter out dey, Rach! I'm s'pose tah be his *wife*. I wake up 'n seen all his clothes hangin' 'ney next tah mine in the closet. His shoes lined up jus' so. Nothin' ever out 'a order. Nothin' ever out 'a place. His smell – everywhere. I love it. Love the way it fills up a room. The way it fills me up. But every moment since I found that picture – called that number –

RACHEL. Jesus Christ, Neekie, this is a Jersey number! You did NOT come up here to – You have GOT to be kidding me.

MONIQUE. You thank she pretty? Pretty enough tah leave home fah?

RACHEL. Neekie...?

MONIQUE. Okay. Okay. Listen tah me! Listen tah me please. I'm not stayin'. We jus' need a place tah crash fah a coupla nights til I figure some stuff out. That's it. I ain't askin' fah no money this time. Just...a place tah stay a coupla nights.

RACHEL. You just gonna make trouble for yourself, Neekie. And I don't want to be pulled into no mess / over this.

MONIQUE. Ain't no mess! Ain't no mess, Rachel. Promise.

RACHEL. Baby, if he's *here* with this...this *woman* / there's bound to be –

MONIQUE. You know my baby can't sleep? She loses her breath. Don't speak hardly since her daddy lef' her! Them two? They was in lock-step, man. Me 'n her? We kinda...well, she ain't close tah *me* like she been wit' *him*, ya know. So, she don't tell me much. But that little girl done gone through some hell.

   (Beat.)

On the ride up sure, ya know, all I could thank about was what that woman's face must look like outside 'a that picture. Who she is. Her body –

RACHEL. Jesus...

MONIQUE. But, ya know, I'm *this* close tah seein' this woman's face –

RACHEL. Neekie –

MONIQUE. I'm this close –

RACHEL. Neekie –

MONIQUE. I'm this close 'n nah I really don't think I can do it is what I'm tryna tell ya!! I don't know if I even *want to* anymo'. I jus' need – tah feel – "okay." Safe. Just fah a lil while. Please? Look, the man is gone! I *want* him gone. I want him gone from me. Ain't no need lookin' for somebody don't want to be found. Right? *(Forcefully.)* Right?

RACHEL. Sure but –

MONIQUE. Ain't worth the search. I ain't looking. You ain't looking. Ain't nobody lookin' for Reggie.

RACHEL. *(Reluctantly agrees.)* Ain't nobody looking.

MONIQUE. Jus' a coupla nights?

(Beat.)

RACHEL. We can set up a place for you in the office and Sam can stay out here and sleep on the couch I s'pose.

MONIQUE. It'll jus' be fah a lil while, Rach. Promise.

RACHEL. Don't worry 'bout it.

MONIQUE. Thank you, Rachel. Shouldn't you consult ya better half?

RACHEL. What she gon' say? You here. And contrary to your belief she does have a heart. That beats real blood. And she loves Sam. There's even a little space in there for you too. / You *push* her!

MONIQUE. Mm.

RACHEL. Don't do it while you're here.

MONIQUE. I won't. I promise. It'd jus' be fah a lil while.

RACHEL. However long you need.

MONIQUE. It'd be good fah Sam tah be away from Vixten fah a minute too.

RACHEL. God. Poor baby.

MONIQUE. She'll be fine.

> *(Crosses to the window to peek at* **SAM.***)*

This'll be good. This'll be real good fah her. An' she can catch up wit' her favorite auntie!

RACHEL. Her *only* auntie. Yeah, I'd like that too.

MONIQUE. An' *we* can catch up?

RACHEL. Mm hm.

MONIQUE. An' you right. I ain't gonna push Dima.

> *(Beat.)*

Oh, see nah I hate I had to come up here like this. I wish it could have been fah like ya birthday or Christmas or somethin'.

RACHEL. You come whenever you need to, baby.

MONIQUE. Ohhh, girl!

RACHEL. What?

MONIQUE. THAT'S what we fidnah' do! I'm 'bout make that kitchen sang a lil bit. Can I do that fah ya? Can I make you a Christmas dinner?

RACHEL. You're insane.

MONIQUE. Imma go to the store, come back 'n cook us up a big ole Vixten style meal! How do a pot roast, collard greens, black-eyed peas, rice, cornbread, 'n peach cobbler sound?

RACHEL. *(She holds up her hands in Hallelujah praise. Whispering.)* Better than quinoa.

MONIQUE. Ken who?

(They laugh.)

Rach, Thank you.

RACHEL. Yeah, well, don't thank me yet...

Scene Two

(Brooklyn. Same day. Just outside the brownstone. **SAM** *sits on the stoop. She takes the crackers from the fold of her dress, crushes them tightly in the palm of her hand then studies the crumbs as she allows them to escape through her fingertips. As she does, in the distance, lights slowly rise on the* **GRAVEDIGGER**. *He sits just as she does. Then...)*

REGGIE. *(Sings brightly.)*
Oh, this little piggy say I wan' some corn...

(She runs to him gleefully. Laughing. And suddenly lights are fully up on father and daughter in Vixten, Georgia. The recent past.)

Get on up here, baby girl!

*(**SAM** sits on **REGGIE**'s knee. He holds her by the back of her shirt. As he bounces her, she clumsily dips from side to side. She laughs wildly.)*

(Sings.)

Oh, this little piggy say I wan' some corn
Danky danky dank
Dank dank

I don't know where to get it from
Danky danky dank
Dank dank

Say, this little piggy say I wan' some corn nah
Danky danky dank
Dank dank

I don't know where to get it from

Danky danky dank

Dank dank

Danky danky dank

Dank dank

Ha. See, you like that right d'ere hunh?

> *(He lifts her off of his knee. Massages his thigh.)*

You gettin' so big. You gettin' too big fah me tah put you on my knee, girl.

SAM. That ain't true!

REGGIE. It is too.

SAM. Who say I'm big?

REGGIE. 'Ccording to my leg 'n my back, baby girl.

SAM. Yesterday, I put my whole self in the dryer 'n I spun on the inside of it. If I can fit in a dryer I can fit on yo knee. So 'dey!

REGGIE. "So d'ere" hunh?

SAM. Yeah.

REGGIE. Well, I guess you tol' me!

SAM. I sho did. I ain't too big.

REGGIE. See 'dey, you just bidin' ya time. You is big, Sam.

> *(Beat.)*

Come here, lemme talk tah ya serious. *(Serious business.)* You got 'bout couple more years fah ya gonna start gettin' a lil height on ya. Start worryin' 'bout ya hair 'n clothes 'n ya gonna start... well, ya gonna start growin' them thangs up top d'ere...

SAM. Tittiebones?

REGGIE. Yeah them.

SAM. I know. I know all about 'em. Keisha, girl in my homeroom, she gettin' hers.

REGGIE. You talk to Keisha 'bout it?

SAM. Yeah. She say they hurt when she catch a ball.

REGGIE. You know, I was a awful kid. Somebody tol' me tittiebones hurt girls 'n I usta run up tah 'em an smack 'em square on the ches'.

SAM. That's mean, daddy. Why you did that? That's mean!

REGGIE. I know it was. But see, I was jus' a boy. An' that's what lil boys is sometimes. Stupid lil niggas wit nothin' better to do 'cept make girls cry. It was funny tah me.

SAM. Don't be smackin' *my* tittiebones!

REGGIE. I-I'm not gonna be smackin' yo tittiebones. Trust me.

SAM. I'll bus' you up, man!

REGGIE. Who you gonna bus'?

SAM. You! 'N anybody gonna be smackin' my tittiebones.

REGGIE. Alright. Alright, lil girl ain't nobody messin' wit' you.

SAM. Better not!

REGGIE. An' another thang that's gonna happen ya gonna get ya monthly.

SAM. Monthly what?

REGGIE. Ask ya mama.

SAM. I don't wanna ask her. She don't be talkin' right no way...

REGGIE. *(With softness.)* I know.

SAM. *(Timidly.)* She be mumblin'. I don't understand her sometimes. People be sayin' she stupid.

REGGIE. Who say that?

(**SAM** *averts her eyes.*)

Sam, look at me. Who in the hell be sayin' that 'bout ya mama?

SAM. I don't know! People –

REGGIE. Look here, I don't care who they is. If it's someone big like me or one 'a ya lil friends, Keisha or whoever, don't you ever let nobody talk down 'bout ya mama! You hear me?

SAM. But she don't talk right –

REGGIE. (*With steel.*) Samantha Barber, I swear 'fore God, you talk down 'bout ya mama you ain't no daughter 'a mine.

(*Silence.*)

SAM. (*Stunned and scared.*) Yes sir.

REGGIE. Nah, I don't wanna hear no more 'bout it. When she come 'round, when she get her mind right you ask *her*. Ask her 'bout ya monthly. You need tah be talkin' tah *her* 'bout these thangs. I can only get ya so far.

SAM. Yes sir.

REGGIE. An' ask her 'bout how ya gonna start tah smell different.

SAM. I don't wanna smell no difference.

REGGIE. Well, ya gonna smell different!

SAM. Why?

REGGIE. Cause that's just how it is. That's how the world work. An' sooner or later them boys 'round here gonna catch hol' tah that smell 'n be knockin' on that door.

SAM. What they wanna smell me fah?

REGGIE. 'Cause that's how boys is. They catch hol' tah a woman scent 'n it be like a dog on a bone. Ain't nothin' a man like better in the world. And ain't nothin' he can do 'bout it neither.

SAM. Boys ain't got nothin' better tah do than smell girls? Make 'em cry? That's dumb.

REGGIE. Boys *is* dumb! But they'll be changin' too. Right 'long witcha.

SAM. They gonna smell difference?

REGGIE. Yeah. It won't be sweet though. But you find one ya won't mind the smell of 'ventually.

SAM. An' they'll have they monthly?

REGGIE. Boys don't have no monthly, girl! How you know 'bout tittiebones 'n don't know 'bout monthlies?

SAM. Keisha ain't said nothin' 'bout no monthly! Just tittiebones! Boys don't get 'em?

REGGIE. No! An' I don't want ya talkin' tah no damn Keisha no mo. She sound fast. Ya don't need tah be hangin' 'round no fast girls. You ask ya mama from now on 'bout women stuff, ya hear me?

(**SAM** *nods yes.*)

(*Beat.*)

SAM. Why not?

REGGIE. Why not what?

SAM. Boys don't get no monthly. Why not?

REGGIE. Cause they boys! That's just the way thangs is, girl. You get bigger. You starts to fill out. You ain't gonna take no more rides in the clothes dryer or on ya daddy knee. Boys be wantin' tah come 'round here 'n smell you 'n take you away.

SAM. I ain't goin' noway.

REGGIE. By the time they come 'round askin' fah ya, you gonna wanna go. Trust me.

SAM. I ain't gonna smell no difference! I ain't gettin' no bigger! An' I ain't goin' noway! You can forget it, man! I guess I *tol'* you!

> (**REGGIE** *can't help it. He's proud of this kid he's raised. Smiles.*)

REGGIE. I reckon ya did.

> (**SAM** *laughs but the sound of heels on pavement disrupts her. As the lights fade on* **REGGIE** *so does* **SAM***'s smile. And at once, we are back in Brooklyn.* **SAM** *turns to see* **NADIMA** *approaching – a canvas bag of groceries in one arm while on the phone.*)

NADIMA. *(Into the phone.)* Hey. Hold on. *(To* **SAM**.*)* You're not banished, ya know. It's nice in there too.

> (**SAM** *says nothing.* **NADIMA** *smiles and gives* **SAM** *a soft pat on the cheek.*)

Huh. Okay, kiddo. Suit yourself.

(Into the phone.) Gary? I'm back.

Scene Three

*(**NADIMA** enters the apartment continuing her conversation. Heads into the kitchen.)*

NADIMA. But see that's what pisses me off – You should have *told* me the homeowner wanted to see a draft of the project by Monday. Well, it doesn't mean that it's going to happen. If you – Hold on –

(Takes out food. "Kids" food. Fruit. Organic this. Kale Chips. Stuff kids hate actually.)

Because of the damn wall! If it's weight bearing – Yeah. Yeah. Yeah. Exactly. If not? If not then, *(In her best Faye Dunaway as Joan Crawford.)* "Tear down that *bitch* of a bearing wall and put a window where it *ought* to be!!"

(Beat.)

Jesus, Gary you are an embarrassment to gay men everywhere. *Mommy Dearest.*

(She heads into the office.)

Don't *ask* him, Gary. *Tell* him. You're the project manager. Aggh!!

(Runs out of the office. Mortified.)

Gary, let me call you back. Just why! Why!

*(**MONIQUE** emerges from the office in a robe. Obviously fresh from a shower.)*

MONIQUE. I was tol' I could use the office / as my –

NADIMA. The HORROR of what I just saw.

MONIQUE. Oh, shut d'hell up! An' be quiet.

NADIMA. Nightmarish.

MONIQUE. Sam *still* out dey...

> (**NADIMA** *sucks her teeth. Crosses to the window. Peeks out at* **SAM**.)

NADIMA. She knows she can come in, right? I told her as much.

MONIQUE. Too much excitement outside I s'pose...

NADIMA. Bought her some snacks. Does she like kale chips?

MONIQUE. What's that?

NADIMA. A little salty. A little crunchy.

MONIQUE. I'm sure she'll like 'em. Thank you. You bought me a snack?

NADIMA. *(Eyeing her rather coldly but playfully.)* I guess you can eat some too.

> (**NADIMA** *enters the kitchen.*)

MONIQUE. Well, ain't you jus' the sweetest thang that ever was.

(*Calling to* **NADIMA**.) Hey, y'all been tah all these places?

NADIMA. Where's that?

MONIQUE. All these places on y'alls wall?

NADIMA. *(Entering with chips.)* Not really.

> (*Looks at a picture. Laughs a little.*)

Hmph.

MONIQUE. What?

NADIMA. Nothing just... Do you know what staging is? Never–[mind]... It's... I doll up these dinky properties out in Canarsie with bits of furniture and photos...that I print myself. Saves money. Hanging them up here saves money on storage.

MONIQUE. Oh.

NADIMA. *(Shyly.)* Not that I wouldn't *want* to go. A wish list in photographs. I can't get your scaredy cat sister to leave the States for anything though. Scared of flying. Scared of boats. Scared of anything that gets her from point a to point b. Surprising she made it this far.

MONIQUE. Blame that one on Mama. She wasn't one fah leavin' the house too much no way. Nor the *bed* for that matter. 'Specially after daddy died… Me 'n Rach born into fear. Like brown eyes 'n bad money. Rach did better than me though. She *is* here. Teachin' these lil rude assed kids y'all got up here. I heard jus' 'bout every piece of "f this" and "f that." From kids Sam's age jus' 'bout!

NADIMA. Well, *her* students are college-aged. Pseudo-*intellectual* foul-mouths. But, yeah.

MONIQUE. I don't like that. Kids only ought to have hard candy, sour pickle with a Now 'n Later in the middle of it kinda words. Not dis here.

NADIMA. Well, what can you do? They're not yours and you can't smack 'em around, you know.

MONIQUE. *(Carefully.)* You – you think you'd smack yo kids? I was spanked 'n all but I don't do that wit' Sam.

NADIMA. *(Laughs.)* Oh god! Ha. You're asking the wrong one, honey. Sam's a good kid though. So…

MONIQUE. Yeah.

NADIMA. Barcelona. That's where I wanna start. *(Rubs her temples.)* If I can just get this *next* place finished? We are…starting in Barcelona. Then Sicily. Down to Egypt. Maybe you can convince Rach to go a little further east than Riis Beach for me?

MONIQUE. Hunh. I couldn't even convince her tah make a detour back down south. You keep my sister locked up or somethin'?

NADIMA. Okay. I don't *keep* your sister from doing anything. You want to talk about the time that's gone by between the two of you seeing each other? Take it up with your sister. She's chain free.

MONIQUE. Hmph.

NADIMA. And we *have* come down, Monique!

MONIQUE. For like *one* weekend a hundred years ago! Flew in 'n outta 'dey like a passin' breeze. She's missin' most of Sam growin' up –

NADIMA. And whose fault is that? Really. You know, it's hard to visit chaos. And that, on *top* of sending part of your savings / every time there's an emergency.

MONIQUE. *(Ending it.)* I promised Rach I wasn't gonna push ya buttons. Let me shut up.

(Beat.)

I am gonna find me some pictures 'n make *me* a wish list wall 'a all the places I wanna go too. Bike week. Bronner Brothers. Essence Fest.

(She laughs hard and loud. Like she needed it.)

NADIMA. *(Laughs. Offering a chip.)* Here.

MONIQUE. They green.

NADIMA. It's Kale. Kale's green.

MONIQUE. What's that on 'em?

NADIMA. Sesame seeds.

MONIQUE. You jokin' right?

NADIMA. About?

MONIQUE. You thank a kid gonna eat that mess? Man, get that shit from 'round me.

NADIMA. You're right. I wouldn't expect for you to have an open mind or to try something new.

MONIQUE. It's fried at least?

NADIMA. No.

MONIQUE. Then how it crisp –

NADIMA. Just TRY it.

>   (**MONIQUE** *smells it. Then nibbles on it. She likes it. She refuses to let* **NADIMA** *know, however.*)

MONIQUE. Taste like collard greens! Why would they *make* somethin' like that?

NADIMA. (*Pleased with herself seeing that she's won.*) See, that didn't kill you.

MONIQUE. It ain't went all the way down yet. We'll see.

NADIMA. If that doesn't work I have a hammer under the sink.

MONIQUE. See, why you gotta act like that?

NADIMA. Like?

MONIQUE. Rude. Ain't nobody want nothin' from you!

NADIMA. Besides room and board.

MONIQUE. We ain't stayin' long.

NADIMA. So you've said.

MONIQUE. (*Sucks her teeth. Under her breath.*) Man, fuck you.

NADIMA. I'm sorry. What was that?

MONIQUE. (*In a mockingly sweet southern style.*) Much obliged, ma'am. We be right out from under your hair directly. Promise, boss lady. Wouldn't want us field niggas come mess up y'alls great big ole fine Big House wit' our poor lil ole nasty ass presence 'n shit.

(**NADIMA** *turns to* **MONIQUE** *and suddenly pulls at* **MONIQUE**'s *arm and struggles to release it from her side.* **MONIQUE** *fights her but finally succumbs.* **NADIMA** *turns* **MONIQUE**'s *arm to reveal needle tracks, some newer than others.*)

NADIMA. You are a piece of work. Why are you here?

MONIQUE. Let go 'a me.

NADIMA. Seriously, what the hell *else* could you possibly want from Rachel?

MONIQUE. I ain't asked her / for nothin'!

NADIMA. I don't want that shit in my house.

MONIQUE. I ain't got nothin' wit' me.

NADIMA. Look at me. Look at me!

(**MONIQUE** *does.*)

You don't have anything with you?

MONIQUE. I said no!

NADIMA. Not even something to tide you over?

(**MONIQUE** *quiets.*)

That's the last of it, Monique. Don't find it in this neighborhood or anywhere near here. Am I making myself clear?

MONIQUE. How you talk tah me like that?! I'm a grown ass woman! / You can't be talkin' to me –

NADIMA. Then act like one!

I don't want it in my house, Monique!

MONIQUE. This my sistah house too 'n I'm stayin' wit' her. Not you! Nah, turn me loose, you big ole greasy bulldagger!

(**RACHEL** *enters undetected with more bags of groceries just as "bulldagger" escapes from* **MONIQUE**'s *lips.* **SAM** *at her side.*)

NADIMA. *(Laughs.)* What the fu–? Okay. "Bulldagger"? Always got your hand out. Calling me names with your goddamn hand out and your mouth *wide* open.

(*She grabs her a little more roughly.*)

I am *this* close to –

RACHEL. There's my girls!

(*The* **WOMEN** *are frozen for a bit. Beat. A terse* **RACHEL.**)

Dima, help me with these bags please. Thank you.

(**MONIQUE** *stares at* **NADIMA** *who finally releases her grip and crosses to help* **RACHEL** *with the bags. They see* **SAM** *who eyes her mother coldly. Under their breaths.*)

MONIQUE. Shit.   **NADIMA.** Dammit.

RACHEL. *(To* **MONIQUE.***)* You know whatever you call her you call me? You know that right?

MONIQUE. Rach, you know I –

RACHEL. Whatever you call her you call me.

(**MONIQUE** *hangs her head. A moment.*)

Remember where you are, what you need and who you're asking it from.

MONIQUE. I will.

RACHEL. *That* side of Vixten is the reason why *this* is my home now.

(*Beat.*)

Okay, did I hear an apology?

MONIQUE. I was just / tryin' tah tell her...

RACHEL. To *both* of us.

MONIQUE. *(Mumbles.)* I'm / sorry.

NADIMA. *(Waving off the apology dismissively. Still heated.)* Ahh don't even...

RACHEL. *(Giving **NADIMA** a stinging look. To **MONIQUE**.)* You better put some clothes on if you gonna be cookin' this here food.

NADIMA. I brought home groceries.

RACHEL. Christmas dinner? No, you did not.

NADIMA. Christmas dinner?

MONIQUE. *(Sheepishly.)* I'm making y'all a Christmas dinner tonight. To say thank you...

RACHEL. *(A forced smile.)* She sho is.

MONIQUE. And Sammie's gonna help. Ain't you, baby?

*(**SAM** storms back out the apartment.)*

Baby! Shit...

(Beat.)

*(**RACHEL** tosses a grocery bag on the ground in frustration.)*

RACHEL. Oh, y'all I am too too too excited for this here dinner!

MONIQUE. I'm sorry, Rach. Imma fix it. Imma fix all of it.

(Beat.)

(Re: The groceries.) I said I was gonna go tah the store.

RACHEL. With what money?

MONIQUE. I was gonna get –

RACHEL. *(Suppressing her rage.)* You was gonna pay for all of the food *and* cook it? No ma'am. It's the least I could do.

MONIQUE. I'm sorry, Rach. I'll –

RACHEL. Go on and get dressed and get your baby from outside. It's too dark for her be sittin' out there stewin' like that. Go on.

> (**MONIQUE** *does as she's told. The couple exchange glances that read* **RACHEL**: *"I can't believe you"* / **NADIMA**: *"What?"* **RACHEL** *enters the kitchen pissed.* **NADIMA** *is alone for a guilty awkward moment.* **RACHEL**, *having taken a breath, returns from the kitchen and stands square to* **NADIMA**.)

NADIMA. *(Gently starts toward* **RACHEL**.*)* Baby...have you seen your sister's arms? There's only so much I'm willing to –

RACHEL. *(Still trying to calm down.)* One second.

NADIMA. Sure.

> *(Beat.* **NADIMA** *sits.* **RACHEL** *pointed. Fierce.)*

RACHEL. High school. Okay? We would drive around town in circles at nights over the weekend. Or sometimes just up the road and back down it again. Cruisin'.

NADIMA. *(Carefully.)* Okay –

RACHEL. And that was Friday night and Saturday night. And the *next* Friday and the *next* Saturday. 'Cause that's all that was left for us to do. Other than that, kids were bored shitless. But, there are two even better things that *really* save you from boredom in a small town. My sister has been thoroughly entertained by both. And now, the plant's not even there to hold that raggedy ass town together and Reggie's gone off with someone else.

That is what has knocked her on her side, broken up her family, and what her little girl has to look forward to.

NADIMA. I get it.

RACHEL. Good. And sweetie, if you lay another hand on my sister, you don't ever have to worry about me walking through that door again.

> *(**NADIMA** looks at **RACHEL** in disbelief. Then, meticulously grabs her keys, phone, and jacket. **RACHEL**, stunned by the weight of her own words, can only watch as **NADIMA** exits the apartment.)*

SAM. *(On the stoop. Trying to calm herself.)*
Down Down Baby Down by the rollercoaster
Sweet Sweet Baby, I'll never let you go…

> *(**NADIMA** looks at **SAM** and out into the night. Pats her on the head.)*

NADIMA. Be right back.

> *(As **NADIMA** exits, **SAM**'s breathing quickens.)*

Scene Four

> (**SAM**, *on the brownstone stoop, tries to calm her breathing. And, from inside the apartment, a still-stunned* **RACHEL** *is doing the same.* **SAM** *closes her eyes.*)

SAM.

Down Down Baby Down by the rollercoaster
Sweet Sweet Baby, I'll never let you go...

> (*Breath. She pulls at the hem of her dress.*)

Shimmy shimmy cocoa puff shimmy shimmy I
Shimmy shimmy cocoa puff shimmy shimmy I

> (*As she sings* **REGGIE** *and* **MONIQUE** *appear. Vixten, Georgia, back in the day. They are younger than we've seen them. Him fifteen. Her fourteen. The way they drape themselves hides* **MONIQUE***'s body somewhat.* **SAM** *opens her eyes.*)

I like coffee I like tea
I like a black boy 'n he like me
So step back white boy you don't shine
I'll get a colored boy to beat ya behind

> (**SAM** *takes a deep breath and looks at them longingly. Lights fade on* **SAM** *and* **RACHEL** *in Brooklyn as* **REGGIE** *and* **MONIQUE** *linger sweetly off of a romantic R&B hit. Something in the vein of "Into You" by Fabolous and Ashanti.**)

---

* A license to produce *Last Night and the Night Before* does not include a performance license for "Into You." The publisher and author suggest that the licensee contact ASCAP or BMI to ascertain the music publisher and contact such music publisher to license or acquire permission for performance of the song. If a license or permission is unattainable for

REGGIE. Moon happy tonight. Lit up almost like daytime. Shinin' fah you, girl.

MONIQUE. You just full a' songs 'n poems, boy.

REGGIE. I write *you* a poem. Write one like ya used tah write.

MONIQUE. Oh yeah? Write me a poem then. What it say?

REGGIE. Damn, girl. You look so fine. You look so fine in the Moonlight, girl. Bright jus' like you, baby.

MONIQUE. That's *game*, fool. That ain't no damn poetry. That's some playa shit.

REGGIE. No, it ain't neither!

MONIQUE. Bullshit.

REGGIE. Bullshit hunh? You gonna have enough of bullshittin' the Moon, girl. Moonlight don't play! The Moonlight mean somethin' bigger, girl. Like…see how I compare ya tah the Moonlight? When I see you in it? Ya know what that mean?

MONIQUE. What?

REGGIE. You shine in the darkness.

MONIQUE. Mm hm.

REGGIE. You light up. I see thangs clearer when you around.

MONIQUE. Do ya now?

REGGIE. Yeah. Like when it get dark 'n the Moon's up d'ere? It's a little bit 'a hope. Hope ain't no bullshit.

MONIQUE. Hope sound like game tah me.

REGGIE. Call it what you wanna, female. But Imma tell ya like this again. Don't be bullshittin' no Moon.

"Into You," the licensee may not use the song in *Last Night and the Night Before* but should create an original composition in a similar style or use a similar song in the public domain. For further information, please see the Music and Third-Party Materials Use Note on page iii.

MONIQUE. Why? What'll happen if I do?

REGGIE. Woman, you liable tah make the seas change course! You liable tah hurt its feelings 'n have it run away.

> (**MONIQUE** *laughs.*)

Have the sun out all day 'n burn us to ashes. You wanna be ashes?

MONIQUE. No, I do not wants tah be no ashes thank you.

REGGIE. *(To the moon.)* See! No ashes fah *my* baby! No thank you.

Nah, tell the Moon ya sorry.

MONIQUE. Man, you crazy. I ain't –

REGGIE. Woman, you best 'pologize tah the Moon. I told ya what was liable tah happen nah!

MONIQUE. *(Reluctantly, but just in case.)* Nah look here, Moon. You know I was jus' playin' right.

REGGIE. I'm sssss–

MONIQUE. I'm sorry, Moon. D'ere. Satisfied? *(Sucks teeth. Laughs.)* You so stupid.

> (**REGGIE** *takes* **MONIQUE**'s *hand. He rocks* **MONIQUE** *slowly. Touches her just heavy pregnant belly. Gently and with subtle desperation.*)

REGGIE. See, it's workin' ain't it? I told ya it would, Neekie. You been doin' real good these last couple months.

MONIQUE. It is workin'. A *lot*. I feel…clearer. Lighter. I do. I hope it stick.

REGGIE. It will.

> *(Smiles with a bit of self-congratulation.)*

We ain't got no other choice, right?

MONIQUE. Right.

(A pensive sadness.)

You look so happy.

REGGIE. Can't a nigga grin? Shit.

MONIQUE. I ain't sayin' you can't! Shit.

REGGIE. Let a nigga grin den! Shit.

(He laughs. Beat.)

You happy *too* though ain't ya?

MONIQUE. *(Uncertain.)* Yeah. Yeah. I'm kinda workin' on somethin' new too. / So…I guess it *is* workin'.

REGGIE. *(Excited.)* Owwww / sheeeet!

MONIQUE. *(Playfully.)* Now, it's not as good as *your* little piece 'a poetry but –.

REGGIE. For real? Whatca holdin' back fah then, woman! Show me how it's done.

MONIQUE. Now, I'm *workin'* on it…

REGGIE. Don't care. Talk tah me, female.

MONIQUE. Okay! Okay so… It ain't much but I think it go… I think it go…

Startled intah creation

Shifted awake

From an imagination

Turn't loose

Onna existence

Tah brighten…

(Correcting herself.)

Tah *enlighten*…

See, dat's the word I ain't got yet.

MONIQUE. Tah enlighten...

(Suddenly finding the word she needs.)

Tah shore up!
Tah shore up
A weary worl'.
A would-be Griot
Begets a' unnamed Guide
Uncertain of the terrain.
They,
As if sewn from fabric made 'a
History's skin,
Walk in tandem
Prayin' pitfalls are shallow
And Masters have mercy on rebellious slaves.

(Silence.)

REGGIE. Damn.

(Beat.)

What that mean?

MONIQUE. Don't worry 'bout it.

REGGIE. Girl, you a powerful somethin' else! Powerful. Writin' all smart 'n whatnot. You seen what else you jus' did? Savin' the world from a upset Moon?

MONIQUE. What's that?

REGGIE. You done made it safe fah my lil man tah come into d'world. You done set it up right fah 'im.

(They move together to the music.)

Scene Five

(The sweet R&B jam makes way for an upbeat Soulful Christmas classic in the vein of "This Christmas" by Donny Hathaway.* Brooklyn. Dinnertime. **SAM**, *still done up in her dress, enters with a box of Christmas décor. She starts to place lights and figurines from the box around the space. Her heart slowly warming to whatever holiday magic she can conjure from them and the music. She finds and holds onto a Black Santa Elvis doll.)*

*(***RACHEL*** enters. Dressed up for the occasion. She helps* **SAM** *who accepts her assistance with ease.)*

*(***MONIQUE*** – dressed up as much as she can be [maybe a borrowed shirt] – enters with a tiny Christmas tree and playfully engages* **SAM** *with it.* **SAM** *gives her the cold shoulder. Still resistant to her mother's efforts. The music fades and...)*

(As the sisters continue to fuss about with decorations and setting the table, **NADIMA** *– dressed casually – enters from the bedroom.)*

---

* A license to produce *Last Night and the Night Before* does not include a performance license for "This Christmas." The publisher and author suggest that the licensee contact ASCAP or BMI to ascertain the music publisher and contact such music publisher to license or acquire permission for performance of the song. If a license or permission is unattainable for "This Christmas," the licensee may not use the song in *Last Night and the Night Before* but should create an original composition in a similar style or use a similar song in the public domain. For further information, please see the Music and Third-Party Materials Use Note on page iii.

NADIMA. *(Wrly.)* A crisp cool eighty-five-degree day? Sure, this totally makes sense.

MONIQUE. Ain't nobody studyin' you. *(To* **RACHEL**.*)* How dat look?

RACHEL. Everything looks delicious, Neekie.

MONIQUE. I hope it taste all right. The decorations?

NADIMA. Where'd you find all this stuff?

RACHEL. Y'all went all OUT!

MONIQUE. Y'alls basement.

NADIMA. You went down there? By yourself?

SAM. I went too! Mama was scared, so I went in first.

RACHEL. She speaks!

NADIMA. It's a Christmas Miracle! That was very brave, Sam. No one's been down there since...

RACHEL. Since our first Christmas together?

NADIMA. That's what I mean.

> (**RACHEL** *crosses to* **NADIMA** *with trepidation. Playfully nudges her. The beginnings of an apology.*)

RACHEL. Nadima tried to impress me when we first got together. We met 'round the holidays –

NADIMA. We don't have to –

RACHEL. I was going on and on about how Christmas was my favorite time of year and-and how I was gonna be away from my family *again* so – Ha! It was so sweet – this woman went buck wild in the ninety-nine-cent store, y'all! Christmas exploded up in this house! Snowflakes on the walls. Had that little ole fake Christmas tree...

(**SAM** *runs across the room. She turns on the Christmas tree.*)

SAM. I think it's nice.

NADIMA. *(Grins.)* Eh.

RACHEL. That string of lights with every color of the rainbow. Cheap as you please.

(**SAM** *runs to plug the lights in. When they are connected, they light up the arch of the doorway.*)

SAM. Tada!

RACHEL. Gorgeous! Simply gorgeous, baby.

MONIQUE. You did all that for my sister?

NADIMA. I was raised by a couple of radical intellectuals who reasoned the "Holiday Spirit" out of everything. So, I don't know, I just took a stab at it. An eccentric stab. *(Smiles.)* It paid off.

(**RACHEL** *wraps her arms around* **NADIMA** *who leans into the embrace.*)

RACHEL. She had this place lit up from night til dawn with holiday music, lights and a very very special elf costume for Christmas night I might add. *(Laughs.)*

NADIMA. *(Laughs.)* Okay!

MONIQUE. Why you 'shamed of that? Ain't nothin' to be 'shamed of.

RACHEL. It was very romantic. And the biggest-hearted thing anyone had ever done for me.

(**RACHEL** *taps her own lips for* **NADIMA** *to kiss.*)

NADIMA. With pleasure.

(They kiss lovingly. In this moment, all is forgiven.)

SAM. Can I see the elf costume?

NADIMA. No, it wouldn't be / something you need to see.

MONIQUE. Imma say no on that one / fah you tonight, Boo.

RACHEL. It may not be appropriate…

(Beat.)

MONIQUE. We should get everyone together.

RACHEL. This is *your* show, baby.

MONIQUE. Okay so y'all, let's gather 'round the table. 'Member how daddy did it, Rach? *(Like Daddy.)* Come on now here youngin' 'n get 'round this here table 'n let's get prayed up real quick like.

RACHEL. Ha! The man was ret' tah eat!

MONIQUE. All the time.

RACHEL. All the time.

*(Finally, the **WOMEN** and **SAM** sit down before a feast of the most delicious-looking southern cuisine you would ever want to see. **MONIQUE** stands. Takes **RACHEL**'s hand in one hand and takes **NADIMA**'s hand with her other. And **SAM** holds her **AUNTIES**' hands in prayer.)*

MONIQUE. Let's bow 'a heads. Lord, we come tah you t'day in prayer so that we may give thanks 'n honor tah you in all thangs. First among those your only begotten son. And also fah the food that you have laid before us. Please bless the hands that have prepared this meal.

SAM. My hands?

MONIQUE. That's right bless my little Sammie's hands 'n let no hurt, harm, or danger come tah us as we share in your bounty. We thank you, Dear Father, fah your design that would have us live another day in your glory. We thank ya also fah the family, Dear God, without whom we could not carry on. We thank ya fah the home you have built. For the roof above 'a heads that we may remain dry when the rains come 'n the foundation on which we stand, fah we know all stability 'n protection comes from you, dear Father. *(Her voice breaks.)* I ask that you wrap your arms around my sister Rachel, Nadima... 'n my lil girl. I ask that ya... *(Starts to tear up.)*

RACHEL. *(Places a hand on **MONIQUE**'s back.)* It's alright, / Neekie.

SAM. Mama?

MONIQUE. I ask that ya give me strength...

*(An excruciatingly long pause as **NADIMA** and **RACHEL** exchange looks. **RACHEL** holds **SAM** close to her.)*

Give me strength tah... We pray all of these things in the name of ya son Christ Jesus. Amen.

RACHEL. Amen.

SAM. Amen.

*(**SAM** looks at her family as they begin to eat. Then, her eyes meet **MONIQUE**'s. Mother picks up a side dish and offers it to her daughter. A peace offering of sorts. But, **SAM** refuses the nourishment. **MONIQUE**'s tearful outburst, to **SAM**, reads as just another hopeful moment tarnished. **SAM** abruptly exits to the office. Leaving **MONIQUE** defeated and guilty.)*

(RACHEL and NADIMA look on as MONIQUE sits embarrassed. And, in a flash, MONIQUE exits, rushing behind her daughter to try and fix what's broken between them.)

(The sound of an oddly bright Christmas Classic similar to Aretha Franklin's "Winter Wonderland" plays as...*)

(RACHEL, helpless, stops just short of rushing to her sister's aid. And NADIMA's heart sinks for her girlfriend. The lights shift. NADIMA carefully comforts RACHEL.)

NADIMA. You good?

RACHEL. Mm.

(RACHEL puts on a brave smile. Then crosses to retrieve bedding from the center chest. NADIMA, holding her concern, clears the table while RACHEL makes her niece's "bed" at the couch.)

(NADIMA re-enters from the kitchen. Watches RACHEL turn off the Christmas lights. Then, crosses to her and pulls her into an easy and playful slow drag to the music. RACHEL laughs and melts into NADIMA. There is lightness here. The lovers sweetly exit into the bedroom.)

---

* A license to produce *Last Night and the Night Before* does not include a performance license for "Winter Wonderland." The publisher and author suggest that the licensee contact ASCAP or BMI to ascertain the music publisher and contact such music publisher to license or acquire permission for performance of the song. If a license or permission is unattainable for "Winter Wonderland," the licensee may not use the song in *Last Night and the Night Before* but should create an original composition in a similar style or use a similar song in the public domain. For further information, please see the Music and Third-Party Materials Use Note on page iii.

Scene Six

(Brooklyn. Late night. The bright Christmas music fades. **SAM** *enters and surveys the living room as if for the first time. She finds the Black Santa Elvis. Picks him up. Grins.)*

SAM. *(Re: Santa Elvis.)* Dis is dumb. *(To Santa Elvis.)* Why you so dumb?

(She likes him. She crosses with him to the window and looks out into the Brooklyn night. Sings/plays this hand game into her new toy.)

Last night and the night before.

I met my baby at the candy store.

He brought me ice cream he brought me cake.

He brought me home with a bellyache.

(As **SAM** *becomes more fixated with Santa lights slowly fade up on* **MONIQUE** *again in Vixten. No longer pregnant. A little older. She starts a slow slump over. A heroin slump.* **MONIQUE** *is in an inebriated remembering of the romantic moonlight of Scene Four.)*

REGGIE. *(Offstage.)* Neekie? Neekie, the baby cryin'...

MONIQUE. *(Incoherent.)* I can't... hol' up. Hol' up a sec.

SAM.
Mama, mama, I feel sick
Call the doctor, quick, quick, quick.

REGGIE. *(Offstage.)* Imma need you tah rock her. 'Kay?

SAM.
Doctah, doctah, will I die?
Close your eyes and count to five
One. Two. Three. Four. Five.

(**REGGIE** *enters. Watches* **MONIQUE**.)

REGGIE. *(Exhausted with bitter sadness.)* Need ya tah feed her. You can't do that?

MONIQUE. You need tah…ya need tah hol' me.

REGGIE. I don't wanna hol' you.

MONIQUE. Hol' me up, Reggie!

REGGIE. What I wanna touch you fah?

MONIQUE. I'm comin'. Jus'… Cause you…you.

> *(She slumps in that slow-motion way again down down down almost into a crouch.)*

REGGIE. *(Screams.)* Ahhh!! *(He moves to her. Forces her to standing.)* Why you do this?! Hunh? Why you do this tah ya'self? *I'm* here. Our baby here! Remember? You don't need this stuff no more.

MONIQUE. You rough, man! *(Incoherent.)* Ya hands all rough on me.

REGGIE. *I'm* here…

> *(He holds her head up. Angrily tries to kiss her. Disgusted.)*

Where's my Neekie?

MONIQUE. I ain't gon' noway.

REGGIE. *(Looks into her eyes.)* Naw you took her someplace! *(Darkening.)* I feel myself dying, Neekie. You need tah 'pologize to the moon, baby. You done wrecked the world.

SAM.
One. Two. Three. / Four. Five.

REGGIE. 'Pologize to the moon, baby! Do it! Do it dammit!

SAM.
One. Two. Three. / Four. Five.

REGGIE. 'Pologize...

> *(As he holds her he is slowly drawn down with her. Her body melts into his frame. He rocks her there slowly.)*

You done wrecked the world, baby.

SAM.

One. Two. Three. Four. Five.

I'm Alive!

> *(The lights fade in Vixten.* **SAM** *in the living room with Dumb Santa Elvis. Looks at Elvis again. Grins.)*

Just dumb. *(Places Santa down. To him.)* Don't go nowhere.

> *(She crosses to the Christmas lights along the archway and turns them back on. Admiring them. Remembering the rare good feelings they brought. She returns to the couch. Picks up Santa Elvis and, as she tucks herself in, she sings to him.)*

See that house on top of the hill?

That's where me and my baby gonna live.

Eat a piece of meat.

Eat a piece of bread.

Come on, baby. Let's go to bed.

> *(After a moment,* **SAM** *is asleep. Dumb Santa Elvis under her arm. The house is quiet. "Not a creature was stirring, not even a mouse" kind of quiet. And then, a tiny break of light seeps through from the office. A* **FORM** *with a satchel over its back and Santa cap on its head sneaks quietly into the living room. Sleigh bells chime softly in the background.*

The **FORM** *checks in on* **SAM**. *Crosses to the table, stuffs some bread and meat into the bag. Quietly checking back then makes its way to the door. Unlocks the top lock. Damn, too much noise!* **SAM** *stirs. The* **FORM** *waits. Unlocks the second lock. Opens the door. Closes it. The sound of sleigh bells in the distance.)*

Scene Seven

(Brooklyn. Next morning. **SAM** *sits on the couch still wrapped in her blanket holding Dumb Santa Elvis tightly. Waiting.* **NADIMA** *sits at the table in her bathrobe and PJs. Christmas décor still arranged. A moment passes.)*

NADIMA. Sammie, does your mom have a cell phone?

SAM. No ma'am. She did once but she ain't pay the bill on it.

NADIMA. Did she talk to you at all, sweetie, when you were on the road? Did she say anything about going somewhere this morning?

*(***NADIMA*** finds a large cardboard box and starts to place Christmas décor into it.* **SAM**, *seeing her –)*

SAM. Oh, don't put that away!

NADIMA. Honey, we've got to take these down now –

SAM. Please! …Don't. Please, Aunt Dima?

*(***NADIMA*** relents. Shakes her head with mild frustration.* **RACHEL** *enters from the office. Photograph in tow.)*

RACHEL. Jersey.

NADIMA. What?

RACHEL. She's in Jersey, honey.

(Hands over the picture to **NADIMA**.*)*

Friend of Reggie's.

SAM. *(Seeing the picture.)* Hey –

NADIMA. *(Ignoring* **SAM.***)* Oh. This is the friend?

RACHEL. Mm.

NADIMA. *(Dials the number.)* I'm calling.

RACHEL. I don't want to be in the middle of it!

SAM. Aunt Rach, / that's –.

NADIMA. *(Ignoring* **SAM.***)* If we have knowledge about someone else's life being in danger we are under some obligation to give them fair warning don't you think?

RACHEL. No. I don't think.

NADIMA. *(She tries the number again.)* It's busy? What is this 1995?

SAM. Aunt Rach, / that's not –!

NADIMA. Still busy.

RACHEL. Your mom went to meet up with someone baby. You want some breakfast?

SAM. No! I ain't hungry!! God!!

NADIMA. *(To* **SAM.***)* Shh.

> *(Into the phone. A deer in the headlights.)*

> Hello? Nadima. Brooklyn. No, I-I-I don't know the Power Play Song of… Wait how much?? Can I guess? Hello?

RACHEL. What just happened?

NADIMA. *(Confused.)* Apparently, I was caller 104?

SAM. Aunt Dima! Listen to me!!

NADIMA. *(To* **SAM.***)* Hold on!

> *(To* **RACHEL.** *Bewildered.)* I never win anything and I was caller 104.

SAM. I'm Sexy and I Know it!!

(Beat.)

NADIMA. *(To* **RACHEL**.*)* Is that an act of defiance? I'm not sure what that is.

SAM. That's the Power Play Song 'a the Day! "I'm Sexy and I Know It."

RACHEL. *(To* **NADIMA**.*)* What? You called a radio station?

SAM. *(Snatching the photo from* **NADIMA**.*)* And *this* is Ms. Frampton!

RACHEL. Okay what?

SAM. Mama said tah bring somethin' wit' me that Imma miss. Imma miss my math teacher Ms. Frampton. So, I brung a picture 'a her. I wrote down that number on the back of the picture.

RACHEL. *(Grabs the picture back.) You* did?

SAM. Cause it was the only piece 'a paper I had! Yesterday on the radio they said the Saturday Power Play Song 'a the Day was gonna be –

NADIMA. I'm Sexy and I Know It...

SAM. I wrote it down cause I knew my mama needed the money. And maybe we could...

(Beat.)

You were caller 104. You missed out Aunt Dima.

RACHEL. *(Panicked.)* Where is your mother?!

NADIMA. Okay. Just take it easy, Sweetheart.

RACHEL. You tell me where the hell she is!

SAM. I don't know, Aunt Rachel! She said we had tah be movin' on.

RACHEL. Where? Here with us? Where?!

SAM. I don't know! I don't know! She just say we movin' on! She ain't say where to! I'm sorry. *(Cries.)* Maybe she heard the song and went to get the money in person... I'm sorry.

(**SAM** *starts to hyperventilate.*)

RACHEL. No no no. Come here. I'm sorry I yelled.

NADIMA. Is she okay?

RACHEL. Go get a paper bag or something!

(**NADIMA** *exits.*)

(To **SAM**.*)* Sit down, baby. Sit down right here. Take deep breaths. Real slow.

(*She tends to* **SAM** *until* **NADIMA** *returns with bag and hands it to* **RACHEL**.*)*

Here take this. Breathe into it. Okay? You forgive me? I'm sorry I yelled at you, honey. It's not you okay?

SAM. I'm sorry.

NADIMA. Just take it easy.

(**SAM** *recovers.*)

You better?

SAM. Yes ma'am.

NADIMA. *(Calmly.)* Okay. Your mom said you were moving?

SAM. Yes ma'am.

NADIMA. Is that all she said? Can you remember if she said she wanted to visit with anyone or that she had business to take care of or anything like that?

SAM. No ma'am. I was sleep most 'a the way.

RACHEL. What about before you left Georgia? Did you see any labels on boxes when you packed up the house?

SAM. *(Puts head down. Diverting her eyes.)* We ain't pack nothin'. We jus' left. Somebody put a paper on our door. Mama said we leavin' cause 'a the paper. She said tah grab thangs Imma miss the most. I grabbed Ms. Frampton. I grabbed one 'a my daddy work-shirts tah sleep in 'n that's it.

NADIMA. Your daddy! Where's he?

RACHEL. Where is Reggie, baby? Do you know?

SAM. We left 'fore he come back from workin' at the plant last night.

RACHEL. *(Her heart sinks.)* Oh... The plant ain't closed down? Your daddy's still working there?

*(**SAM** nods yes. She reads her **AUNT**'s face.)*

NADIMA. *(Seeing **RACHEL**'s heartbreak.)* Rach?

RACHEL. I'm alright.

NADIMA. Rach. We need to get in touch with him.

RACHEL. *(Still in a bit of shock.)* Sam, baby you been in those clothes all morning. You go on and wash up for me?

SAM. *(Sits on the couch. Holds Elvis tighter.)* Imma sit here til she come back.

NADIMA. Sam.

SAM. IMMA SIT HERE TIL SHE COME BACK!

RACHEL. *(Holds **SAM**'s head in hands.)* Sweetie, don't worry. Don't you worry okay?

*(A swelling hollowness washes over **SAM**. **RACHEL** notices it.)*

SAM. *(Pushes **RACHEL**'s hands away. An eerily calm review.)* Don't worry. *Eat* something... I ain't stupid, Aunt Rach.

RACHEL. Honey, just wash up and I'll make you something to – *(Catches herself.)*

SAM. I ain't STUPID!

> *(**SAM** hurls Elvis as hard as she can across the room. Breaking him in half. Storms out of the room. Long beat.)*

NADIMA. *(Shakes her head.)* Ho. Ly. Shit... Huh. Took nearly everything she brought with her. *Except* Sam. Okay. My God.

> *(**RACHEL** is nearly sick to her stomach. Head in her hands.)*

Every time. Every time that woman calls or writes or blinks her eyes she wants something from you. / The *second* she showed up –

RACHEL. *(Almost in a daze.)* How would that look? Me slamming the door in my niece's face, Nadima? *(Suddenly crosses to the office door. Knocks.)* / Sammie?

SAM. Leave me / alone!   **NADIMA.** And you believed her!

RACHEL. So did you!

> *(She knocks again.)*

Sam? / Sam

NADIMA. But I kept my eyes open! That's how reason and heartbreak are supposed to work together. Once you've given every bit of your heart and damn near every bit of your money and there's no real "thank you" or change you start running on fumes, baby! I have been running on fumes with your sister since oh about $4,000 ago. Since about the fifth "Imma get my life together" ago.

RACHEL. Nadima, you have brothers. You completely / understand –

NADIMA. But I don't wipe their asses! There comes a point / when you have to stop –

RACHEL. And you didn't *leave* them when they needed you! So.

   (Beat.)

I taught her how to run away!

NADIMA. *(Exhausted.)* Please, Rachel.

RACHEL. I'm not – I'm not making excuses for her all right! I don't know where my sister is!!

In the world…OR up here! *(Points to her head.)* I mean, I didn't really even know half of what she was going through down there. Still don't! Went off to college and been too concerned with myself since then to even ask.

NADIMA. Rach –

RACHEL. God! And that fucked up little brain of hers… used to be so brilliant.

NADIMA. Is that right?

RACHEL. Yes! Nikki Giovanni brilliant! And I know! I know like right now all you can see is every mistake she's ever made and every penny she ever took from us / but –

NADIMA. Rachel –

RACHEL. when that simple-ass Vixten mentality sets in? Watch out, man! She hated it just like I did, but she couldn't get out. I didn't teach her *nothing* different. I didn't get her out.

NADIMA. Honey, you can feel bad about not taking your sister in while you were in school sure. And hey, you know what? It was kind of a crappy thing to do / but

RACHEL. Thanks / for that.

NADIMA. BUT your sister; that woman who got in a car, stuck her child in it, lied to your face, and left that little girl here, is the one that we are dealing with now. Not that twelve-year-old country mouse you remember.

(**RACHEL** *begins to cry.* **NADIMA** *comforts her.*)

Honey, if you are still holding on to some guilt shit / from the past...

RACHEL. You know what a coward is? Being out and proud, but not...*fightin'* for myself in the face of Vixten's ugliness – of my own *mama's* ugliness toward me. If I couldn't fight for myself, Nadima, how the hell was I s'pose to fight for her?

NADIMA. Oh my god...

RACHEL. Mama had a little spill. Busted her hip. Nothing major. Doctor gave her a *fistful* of pain pills. I mean *fistfuls* after *fistfuls* of 'em. She laid up in that bed missing Daddy and just getting meaner. And numb-er. That was Neekie's first lesson in how to escape. I was the second.

NADIMA. Rachel –

RACHEL. But, hey, I had already settled in on a mission of self-preservation and I...blocked that life out. I blocked my *family* out! And I think it just killed something in her.

NADIMA. You are seriously giving yourself way too much credit, baby! You couldn't fix her then and you most certainly can't now. You can't fix somebody who doesn't even believe they're broken. Just can't. We need to call Reggie.

RACHEL. God. We do...

(**NADIMA** *gets her phone.* **RACHEL** *in sudden focus.*)

But what if we don't?

NADIMA. Call him? Why wouldn't we?

RACHEL. What if we – we um...keep her?

NADIMA. Keep her? And do what with her?

RACHEL. Nadima.

NADIMA. Okay, you've gone from wanting to save your sister to kidnapping her child in like two seconds.

RACHEL. She left her with us, Nadima. She's here.

NADIMA. Reggie doesn't know that! Maybe let's not steal his child?

RACHEL. Nadima, Neekie didn't come all the way up here just to play games. Think about this now! She is running from something! I just think she's in too deep to tell us the truth about it.

NADIMA. Rach, I have had enough of giving her the benefit of the fucking doubt! I don't trust Monique. I don't. I don't think that she has your best interest at heart and I certainly don't think she has her *daughter's* best interest at heart.

RACHEL. You don't know her!

NADIMA. How many times does she have to show you who she truly is before you start to believe her?! No. I'm calling Reggie. I'm not going to raise their child for them off of a whim! They're adults. They can fix this mess themselves.

RACHEL. You've made up your mind?

NADIMA. Yes.

RACHEL. Your house. Your rules.

NADIMA. Stop that.

RACHEL. Whatever you say.

NADIMA. *(Starts to dial.)* My love love love, I am trying my damnedest to take care of this. *(Touches* **RACHEL***'s head.)* And this. *(Touches* **RACHEL***'s heart.)* I am saving you from yourself.

RACHEL. Ohhhh.

NADIMA. And your family.

RACHEL. I. Want. Her! That's final.

NADIMA. What?! Okay-wow! I'm sorry, honey. You're being irrational. Emotional and irrational. She's not... *yours*. And, believe me, I am nobody's mommy. Neither are you. And that is something we've agreed upon. If you –

> *(The office door opens. The* **WOMEN** *wait with anticipation.* **SAM** *enters shyly.)*

SAM. I'm... I'm hungry.

> *(The* **WOMEN** *melt. As the lights fade on the* **WOMEN** *and* **SAM**, **REGGIE** *appears in Vixten. Gravedigger that he is. He methodically cleans a gun. He studies it.)*

REGGIE. Now see you gonna laugh. 'Cause you thank everythang I do is funny. It ain't funny. It's meant tah teach ya. How I speak? That's meant tah teach you too. You get older 'n leave this place...one thing ya gonna remember is the music of ya daddy's voice. The memory 'a what made ya. How ya people survived. An' these little games we play? These little hand games? That's your history too... 'cause ya grandmama sat ya mama down when she was smaller 'n you 'n they played these games 'n had the best time that ever was. Then, ya mama taught me ya know that? Shoot, I ain't wanna learn no little girl games. Imma man! *(Laughs.)* What I look like playin' some little girl hand game! But, then we had you. And I taught you. That's a road map. You ever get lost, you find ya way back home *(Points to his chest.)* from them. Understand? And one way or another... I'll come get you.

> *(As* **SAM** *enters dressed as in the Prologue,* **REGGIE** *places the gun in his back waistband.)*

And now what I got? I got?

> *(Sings.)*

I got the rhythm of the head.
Ding dong. *(Nods head.)*

SAM.
Sho' got the rhythm of the head.
Ding dong. *(Nods head.)*

REGGIE.
Let's get the rhythm of the hands. *(Clap Clap.)*

SAM.
Sho' got the rhythm of the hands. *(Clap Clap.)*

REGGIE.
Let's get the rhythm of the feet. *(Stomp Stomp.)*

SAM.
Sho' got the rhythm of the feet. *(Stomp Stomp.)*

REGGIE.
Let's get the rhythm of the Hot Dog. *(Rolls his body under.)*

SAM. *(Hesitates. A small smile. Then.)*
Sho' got the rhythm of the Hot Dog. *(Rolls her body under.)*

REGGIE & SAM.
Ding dong, *(Clap clap, stomp stomp.)* Hot Dog.
Ding dong, *(Clap clap, stomp stomp.)* Hot Dog.
Ding dong, *(Clap clap, stomp stomp.)* Hot Dog.

> *(**REGGIE** touches her face as **SAM**'s smile fades into a knowing darkness.)*

End of Act One

ACT TWO

Prologue

*(Brooklyn. Time has passed. In the dark of early morning, sounds of African, Caribbean, and hip-hop music meld with Islamic and Jewish prayers and the sounds of traffic. **SAM** sits on the stoop. Same hair as the top of the show, but now in jeans and a t-shirt. She's half Vixten. Half Brooklyn. Mischievous. A layer of street smarts hidden in her sly grin. Filling out the last message in her paper "Cootie Catcher.")*

SAM.

Ain't yo mama pretty

Ain't yo mama pretty

She got meatballs in her titties

She got scrambled eggs between her legs

*(As if **SAM** has conjured her mother up, lights slowly reveal **MONIQUE** in Vixten, Georgia. She is alone. Beautiful. Pregnant. Fourteen again. They are two children coming into their own. **SAM** pockets her pencil, picks a color, and works through her first selection of the "Cootie Catcher.")*

Ain't yo mama pretty

Ain't yo mama pretty

MONIQUE. *(To her belly.)* Startin' tah get nervous 'bout keepin' it all inside. My words tah ya. I 'magine ya can't jus' *hear* the words I'm thankin' but you can oh...you can *feel*...everythang. I thank ya runnin' 'round tryna catch them butterflies floatin' 'n mah stomach. That's why ya be kickin' so much.

>   *(**SAM** picks a number and works her second selection of the "Cootie Catcher." Smiles.)*

SAM.

   Ain't yo mama pretty

   Ain't yo mama pretty

MONIQUE. *(Takes a deep breath. Laughs.)* Ya know ya daddy thank ya gonna be a boy right? Look here, lil baby, if you got plans on comin' outta me bein' a boy you bes' stop that mess right now ya hear me! Need me a lil girl. Be my roll dog! *(Suddenly.)* "Sam..." Mm. Like ya great-grandmama. Samantha. McCloud. Barber. That *stubborn* ole woman...was good. Give ya her name, give ya her backbone maybe...

>   *(Lights slowly rise on **REGGIE** in some dark place in the distance, a duffle bag over his shoulder. He is focused, searching; though the heft of time and a waning hope make up the map of his face now.)*

If you a little girl I thank it'll help me a little more. But we don't wanna find out til ya get here. It's like, "let's just add a little surprise 'n happiness to the room on that day" 'cause... *(Fights back tears.)*

>   *(**REGGIE** takes an audible breath. Closes his eyes. **SAM** picks a number and works her third selection of the "Cootie Catcher.")*

SAM.

   Ain't yo mama pretty

   Ain't yo mama pretty

MONIQUE. We gonna be alright you 'n me. I tell ya this: You ain't *never* gonna go one day wit'out *your* mama huggin' on ya. Not one day wit'out *your* mama tellin' ya how much she love you. 'Cause *I* do, baby. Even though I ain't met ya yet. I love you. *(Laughs. Like* **REGGIE***.)* I love ya like the Moonlight, girl. Ha! And I can't wait fah ya tah get here. I hope ya feel that. I hope ya feel my body tellin' ya the truth 'a that.

> *(The lights slowly fade on* **MONIQUE***. She exits. Daughter and father are left illuminated in space.* **SAM** *closes her eyes. Makes a secret wish then picks her third selection from the "Cootie Catcher" and works through it.)*

SAM.

Ain't yo mama pretty

Ain't yo mama pretty

I took her to a party

She turned around and farted

I asked her why she did it

She turned around and shitted

Ain't yo mama pretty

Ain't yo mama pretty

> *(***REGGIE** *opens his eyes. Adjusts the gun. Wipes it clean.* **SAM** *opens a fold of the "Cootie Catcher" to find her dream hidden inside. She grins hopefully.* **SAM** *exits as the sounds of the city meet those of a more recent past and a faraway train.* **REGGIE** *puts the gun in his waistband. Sits on a crate and rests his head in his hands. Then, breaking through his darkness,* **MONIQUE** *enters hands in pockets and cool. She's seen better days.)*

MONIQUE. Man, is you lookin' fah somebody?

> *(***REGGIE** *looks at his wife with a pain-filled joy.)*

Scene One

(Brooklyn. It is early morning. A school day. A work day. Lights slowly rise on the living room. It has changed. The art has come down and has been replaced by drawings done by a child's hand. The furniture is slightly rearranged. And the space is littered with overcompensation. Toys, books, things eleven-year-old girls love. Rachel's schoolwork is scattered on the table. **NADIMA**, *in her undershirt and maybe her dress pants, sits frustrated on the couch. A makeshift pillow made of her jacket. The sofa's throw as a blanket. It is obvious this is where she slept last night.)*

RACHEL. *(From the kitchen.)* Sam, you 'bout ready for school?

*(**NADIMA** stares ahead, bouncing her foot with anger. After a moment, **RACHEL** bursts through the kitchen, coffee in hand, packing a work bag. Almost ignoring **NADIMA**. She both calls out to **SAM** and considers **SAM** in earshot when she addresses **NADIMA**.)*

I said Sam, you ready? Come on now we gonna be late!

NADIMA. What the hell was locking the bedroom door about?

RACHEL. You think I need to be woken up in the middle of the night? You *see* me right now don't you?

NADIMA. Hmph. Shit. Whatever, Rachel.

RACHEL. Yeah whatever.

Sam! I ain't playin' now! Let's go!

SAM. *(From the bedroom.)* Um… Yes ma'am!

NADIMA. Not like there would have been room for me in the bed *anyway*.

RACHEL. Sam has nightmares, / Nadima!

NADIMA. I know! Shit. I know.

RACHEL. What do you want me to do?

NADIMA. Rachel, you *locked* me out!

RACHEL. Samantha Barber, you got five seconds!

SAM. *(From the bedroom.)* I'm / coming!

NADIMA. For crying out loud, I told you I *had* to be out with my buyers / last night!

RACHEL. Huh. *Had* to.

NADIMA. What do you want *me* to do? It's like you would rather me *stay* gone!

RACHEL. Tell me you wouldn't?

(Beat.)

NADIMA. *(Hurt.)* Jesus, / Rachel.

RACHEL. I'm not interested in doing this with you first thing in the morning, Nadima. Samantha, / this is the *last* time now!

NADIMA. *(To herself. Heartbroken.)* And I'm the asshole. / Again.

> *(**SAM** enters. Wild beautiful hair. Pajama top. Nowhere near ready. Balled up sheets in her hands. Visibly shaken.)*

SAM. I'm... I'm...

RACHEL. What the – You supposed to be ready! We 'bout to leave! What you doin'? Laundry?!

SAM. I think I hurt myself!

*(The **WOMEN** snap to attention.)*

RACHEL. What? Let me see, honey.

*(**SAM** gives the bedding to **RACHEL** who inspects it revealing bloodstains at its center.)*

Oh.

NADIMA. *(Seeing the blood.)* Oh, boy.

*(The **WOMEN** laugh sympathetically.)*

SAM. It's not funny! Imma bleed out. Watch! Then y'all ain't going thank it's funny!

RACHEL. No, it's not funny, baby.

NADIMA. *(Grins.)* Oh, man. Wow. Do we uh…do we have enough stuff?

RACHEL. We should. Maybe not?

NADIMA. I'll run out.

RACHEL. You don't have to.

NADIMA. *(A soft plea.)* I *know*. Come on, Rachel…

*(**RACHEL** concedes.)*

*(**SAM** starts to sit on the couch. **RACHEL** immediately sits her down on the coffee table.)*

*(**NADIMA** grabs her jacket, keys and slips on her shoes at the front door. Turns to **SAM**.)*

Sammie…you uh… I'm proud of you.

SAM. Huh?

NADIMA. Uh cause um… There's a…a lot happening. Are you cramping any?

RACHEL. Go.

(Beat.)

NADIMA. *(To* **RACHEL.***) You* need anything?

(A weighted moment. **RACHEL** *shakes her head.* **NADIMA** *exits.)*

SAM. I thank I'm sick. I can't go tah school today.

RACHEL. *(Still lost a bit in* **NADIMA***'s exit.)* Well, you might miss a couple of your first classes but you have to go to school today. I can't stay home from work.

SAM. How Imma go to school if I'm fixin' tah die?!

RACHEL. *(Softly.)* You're not, Baby. You're not. You are becoming a woman. *(She picks up a sheet.)* What's happening to you right now happens to me and to Aunt Dima and just about every other woman in the world once a month.

*(***SAM** *grabs the sheet from her aunt. Looks into it with fear.)*

SAM. *(Quietly.)* Monthly...

RACHEL. That's right. I think I was thirteen? *(Playfully.)* I thought you'd have at least one more year before she caught you.

SAM. *(Some panic.)* Who caught me?

RACHEL. Your Aunt Flow. But, eleven is about right nowadays I suppose. Now, we are going to soak these sheets a little bit, wash 'em in cold water and they'll be good as new. And as for you –.

SAM. I'm gonna smell different.

RACHEL. Different? Sure. You have to take care of yourself a little differently now. Be careful about a few things. I'll show you. It's nothing you can't handle. Oh, this is exciting! I just got like *really* excited! Are you excited?

SAM. *(Not really.)* Mm.

RACHEL. Girl! You ain't only gonna be *actin'* 'umanish you gwine be an actualized 'uman!

SAM. *(Not thrilled.)* Oh.

RACHEL. And it's wonderful, Sammie. It really is. I know it doesn't look like it right now. Right now, it looks kinda scary and bigger than you and…like you're dying. But you're not. I'll tell you a secret. You, in this moment, have become one of the most powerful entities on the planet. In sync with the moon! And my dear, you are today, at eleven years old, more powerful than any man will ever be. But don't tell the boys at school that. You may not be able to get a date for prom if you let that little factoid loose.

> *(With the mention of "boys"* **SAM** *gets particularly ominous. Something shifts.)*

SAM. *(Eerily calm.)* Boys are gonna knock down the door.

RACHEL. What do you mean?

SAM. Because I smell different nah. As soon as it happens they can tell. It changes 'em. Turns 'em into men.

RACHEL. Who told you that?

SAM. *(Darkening.)* A man catch hold tah that smell 'n he can't let go. It's like a dog wit' a bone.

RACHEL. Ha!

SAM. *(Matter of fact.)* It's not funny, Aunt Rach.

> *(***SAM** *starts to hyperventilate. Two heavy knocks sound from the door. Beat.)*

There's a man at yo door.

Scene Two

(That same school day. **REGGIE**, *in Brooklyn for the first time, sits at the table. The* **WOMEN** *and* **SAM** *watch as he eats, no, devours a full plate of food. It's shocking, greedy, and just a bit more man-ish than this lot is used to. There is a thick and quiet tension in the room. The sound of his fork against the plate is the only noise in the air. After a moment...)*

REGGIE. This somethin' else. What ya call this?

SAM. *(Eyeing her father coldly.)* Leftovers.

RACHEL. Stew chicken.

REGGIE. Naw. Stewed chicken ain't sweet like this. This somethin' different here.

SAM. *(Bitterly with forced respectfulness.)* It's Jamaican.

REGGIE. *(Hearing the bite in* **SAM***'s voice.)* Okay. *(Examines* **SAM** *a bit. Tries to lighten.)* And it's flavored wit' this here banana, or what?

SAM. *(Not giving in.)* That ain't a banana. It's a plant'in.

REGGIE. Plan. Tin. Alright. Alright, baby girl.

*(***SAM** *rolls her eyes at the sound of "baby girl.")*

Ladies, this was mighty delicious. Thank you.

RACHEL. You're welcome.

NADIMA. *(Stingingly.)* You done with that plate?

REGGIE. Uh...yeah. Thank you.

*(***NADIMA** *clears his plate and takes it into the kitchen.)*

Sammie girl, come sit next tah ya father.

*(Unmoved, **SAM** stares at her father with intensity. We hear the sound of a dish being slammed in the sink. **NADIMA** reappears and hangs in the kitchen doorway.)*

REGGIE. Come here nah. What? Don't tell me ya scared 'a me. You scared of ya pa?

SAM. *(She glares at him.)* You scared 'a *me*?

(Beat. This weakens him a bit.)

REGGIE. I missed ya, girl. You missed ya daddy?

SAM. I don't know.

RACHEL. Don't be like that, Sam. Course you missed your daddy, honey.

NADIMA. *(With bite.)* Of course, she did.

REGGIE. Well, ya daddy missed you. Real bad.

(He pulls a wrapped package from his duffle bag.)

I brung you somethin'.

*(**SAM** takes the package and tosses it on the table.)*

SAM. If you miss me then why you ain't come get me?

REGGIE. Uh... baby girl... Sam. Thangs like that takes time.

SAM. *(Stern.)* Mama got here inna day. Why it take *you* so long?

REGGIE. After ya mama 'n you left I had tah handle some thangs. You mad at me?

SAM. Pissed off.

REGGIE. You learned some new words livin' up here.

RACHEL. She grew up a little.

REGGIE. Grew up a lot.

RACHEL. We kept calling you, Reggie.

REGGIE. Y'all makin' it seem like I ain't wanna see my lil girl nah! I tol' ya I had some thangs I needed tah get straight first.

NADIMA. I am so sick of this cryptic shit. What "thangs," Reggie?

REGGIE. Watch how you speak in front of my child!

NADIMA. I've *been* saying what I need to say in front of your child. You're concerned now?

RACHEL. You stopped calling us back.

(*Beat.*)

REGGIE. (*To* **SAM**.) Look how you frown up like that. You got that look like ya mama *down*, man!

SAM. Don't talk about her.

RACHEL. Come on, Sam.

SAM. I don't wanna hear nothin' else 'bout her!

REGGIE. Let her be, Rachel. (*To* **SAM**.) You got thangs tah work out too don'tcha, baby?

(*Beat.*)

I'm here now, Sammie.

RACHEL. What, you think you just gon' take off with her now that you got yourself squared away?

REGGIE. (*To* **SAM**.) Uh… Now look here. I need to talk to ya aunties, baby girl.

SAM. Stop calling me that!

REGGIE. I know you mad. I know you mad at me. That's all right.

RACHEL. Sam, go on to your room.

> (**SAM** *doesn't move. Stares at* **REGGIE**.)

Samantha!

SAM. I hate her.

REGGIE. Sammie –

SAM. You say don't let nobody talk down about her. Don't do this. Don't do that. I don't care no more. I hate her. *(Breath starts to quicken.)* I did *everythin'* you say to do, Daddy! And it don't count for nothin'. I hate her.

REGGIE. *(Weary.)* Don't say that, baby girl.

SAM. *(Breathes.)* I did everythin' you say to do! And I'm up *here*… Why?

RACHEL. Reggie?

> (**SAM** *and* **RACHEL** *stand waiting with resolve. Beat.*)

REGGIE. Monique come home actin' real nervous. She say this man…this man she get her stuff from? She took somethin' 'a his.

NADIMA. Money?

REGGIE. *(He nods yes.)* An' a lil 'a his supply 'parently.

> (**RACHEL**'s *heart sinks.* **NADIMA** *sits.*)

I come home from the plant and seen a…note on the door. Note say I got two days tah leave my house. And it wasn't from the bank…

RACHEL. Jesus.

REGGIE. She owed him a good bit 'a money fah the last couple hits she had 'n couldn't pay him fah *this* one. An' she knew she couldn't get no money outta me fah it. So, she put it in her mind that she could jus' take some 'a the money he got layin' round his place.

NADIMA. My god...

REGGIE. He finds out he got stuff 'n money missin' 'n has a "conversation" wit' her. She tell me he don't *touch* her but...

RACHEL. Where is she?

REGGIE. *(Hesitates.)* Now, *that* I...really couldn't tell ya.

NADIMA. When was the last time you talked to her?

REGGIE. *(Pause.)* Nah look, I didn't know thangs was gonna turn out like they did. It ain't all happened like I planned out.

RACHEL. What the hell is going on, Reggie?

REGGIE. I talked to her 'fore she left Vixten. 'Fore I... 'fore I made them hit the road to come here.

RACHEL. *Made* them?

REGGIE. Just thought...Sam'd be safer livin' up here.

NADIMA. I'm sorry...what?

REGGIE. Trus' me, it ain't all turn out how I *planned* though!

SAM. No! She *tol'* you I wasn't *worth* comin' fah. 'Cause she care more about that STUFF than she do me! / I bet you she did!

REGGIE. Sam!

SAM. *SHE* tol' you to leave me here! And she made us lose our house! She took me away from you! She DON'T love us! It's like she don't even know how to!

REGGIE. That's not true!

SAM. Why she leave me then?!

Why did *you*?

I hate her! I hate her! / I hate her!

REGGIE. Look here, baby girl, d'ere's some thangs ya ain't seein' clear!!

SAM. What I don't see?! Tell me! What I don't see?!

> (**SAM** *stares him down and doesn't take her eyes off of him during the following.* **REGGIE** *crumbles at the sight of her glare.*)

REGGIE. (*Studies his child.*) This man... *He* hurt ya mama. He hurt ya sister, Rach. Made her sick. *He* busted up our whole life ya hear me? Not her.

> (*Beat.*)

Here come this nigga wit' his jeans saggin' half way down his ass, gold tooth grinin'. Never worked a damn day in his life. Talkin' 'bout "this my house now, muthafucker. I got your bitch sprung, been had her sprung *and* now I got yo mutherfuckin' house. How you feel nigga?" He push me. Put his hands on me. Laughin' not *at* me but *through* me. Like I wasn't even 'nere. He stomp around my house lookin' through closets. Throwin' thangs on the floor *I* paid for. Pullin' pictures offa *my* walls. Touchin' *my* memories. Eyin' my wife. My daughter. What *I* do? What do I do?

SAM. (*Shaking her head. Seeing what he sees.*) Daddy?

REGGIE. He watchin' them shakin.' All the time laughin'. He step right into my house makin' hisself at home. He move down the hall...turn his back...an' *I*...

> (**REGGIE** *raises his arm. Curl his finger around an imaginary trigger.* **SAM** *jumps. Covers her ears. Starts to breathe heavily.* **REGGIE** *kneels in front of* **SAM**. *Looks into her eyes.*)

You seein' clearer now, baby girl? You 'member what ya *daddy* done?

(**SAM** *nods yes. Trying to catch her breath. He smiles.*)

An' he wasn't boastin' no mo. He wasn't grinnin'. *That's* how you don't let nobody talk down 'bout ya mama.

SAM. I...

I...can –

(**SAM** *starts hyperventilating.*)

REGGIE. I know it. I know it. Come on, Sammie girl. / Let that go.

SAM. I...I can see him. I see where I –

REGGIE. Put that outta ya mind. That ain't ya memory no more. Let me 'n ya mama hol' on tah it. Ya hear me? *(Calm.)* Hey. Hey. I got the rhythm of the head. Come on now. What I got?

SAM. He got a hole through him.

REGGIE. Come on, Sam.

(*He breathes with her slowly.*)

SAM.

Sho got the rhythm of the head...

REGGIE. Yeah. D'ere ya go. Shake it out. Ding dong. That's not ya memory. I got the rhythm of the head. Shake it out. Ding dong. Ding dong.

SAM.

Sho got the rhythm...

(**REGGIE** *quietly takes her head in his hands as they subtly go through the motions. Ding dong. Clap clap. Stomp stomp.*)

REGGIE. Let me hol' that memory fah you.

(Holds her in his arms. She cries. He kisses her forehead. Rocks her. She is every bit of his little girl again.)

REGGIE. People lookin' for ya pa, baby. I put more 'n a couple thousand miles on a Greyhound. And that ain't no life. That ain't no life for ya, Sammie. *(He looks to* **RACHEL.** *A question.)* You...ya *gotta* stay up here wit' ya aunties okay.

*(***RACHEL** *nods an affirmative to* **REGGIE.** **SAM** *holds on to her father's neck. He pains to release her.)*

SAM. No!

(He walks **SAM** *over to* **RACHEL** *who takes* **SAM** *into her arms.* **NADIMA** *clocks the exchange.)*

I wanna go with you.

REGGIE. Come on, Sammie. **RACHEL.** Come here, baby.

NADIMA. Jesus... *(Beat. Shaking with fear.)* You um...say you don't know where she is?

REGGIE. She... S'posed tah been in a lil rehab house fah women just outside 'a Nashville we foun'. I was gonna come' up here to take her over there after I made sure everythang was straight back home. They ain't have no room fah kids.

NADIMA. You could've told us all of that –.

REGGIE. Well, when you washin' a man's blood offa ya, ya don't tend to thank clear. An' we ain't want y'all mixed up knowin' more than ya needed tah. But, she was s'posed tah wait here fah me. I got that message from y'all sayin' she left here – And... I been lookin' fah her since.

NADIMA. You – You killed a man.

REGGIE. That man kill hisself.

NADIMA. Reggie, loving her is one thing but you *killed* him?

REGGIE. He walked into my house!

NADIMA. Reggie you –!

REGGIE. *(Points to* **SAM**.*)* Look at her! What would you do for her? Tell me.

NADIMA. I –

REGGIE. Look at my little girl. *You* tell me!

RACHEL. Anything.

(**NADIMA**, *speechless, looks at* **RACHEL**.*)*

REGGIE. Anythang. That's right. Any damn thang. D'ere's three thangs I got in this world: Sam, my home 'n my Monique. My home is still mine, my Sam is here 'n nere's only one thang missin.' That man was 'bout tah take all I had. Flick at it like lent off a shiny new suit. Like my life ain't nothin'. What me 'n Neekie built wasn't nothin'! It's everythin'. It may not look like much from the outside in but it was all I had! Sometimes I know Neekie don't treat our life like it's anythang. She don't treat herself like she anythang either.

(Beat.)

I don't know why she left without...

(Beat.)

RACHEL. Go. Find my sister, Reggie.

(**NADIMA** *remains nestled in the doorway as the lights fade around* **SAM**, **REGGIE**, *and* **RACHEL**. *And slowly rise on that same fourteen-year-old pregnant* **MONIQUE** *from the prologue. Vixten, Georgia. Joyous. Smiling.)*

MONIQUE.

Oh, little playmate.

Come out 'n play wit' me.

> *(Breath. Breath. As* **MONIQUE** *sings,* **NADIMA** *makes her way from the doorway nervously touching the things that have made her home a home – a picture here, a memory there. Lights rise on* **SAM** *who climbs the brownstone stoop then sits, knees to chest, looking into the Brooklyn afternoon. Mother and daughter are mirror images of each other.)*

And bring yo dollies three.

Climb up mah apple tree.

Scene Three

(That same Brooklyn afternoon. The brownstone living room. **NADIMA** *sits on the arm of the couch. Waiting for something. Uncertain of what.* **RACHEL** *climbs the stoop and sits with her niece.* **MONIQUE** *continues to sing.)*

RACHEL. Hey, baby.

SAM. *(Quietly.)* Hey.

*(***RACHEL*** holds her for a moment.)*

MONIQUE.
Slide down mah rainbow
Into mah cellar door

*(***RACHEL*** climbs the stairs and enters the brownstone to a weary and maybe newly fearful* **NADIMA**.*)*

And we'll be jolly friends forevah more
One two three four!

(Beat.)

NADIMA. How is she?

RACHEL. A little better.

NADIMA. Yeah?

RACHEL. I don't know. This whole…situation is *mightily* fucked up.

NADIMA. *(Sighs.)* Yes, it is. *(Silence.)* Do you um… do you think she feels *safe?* Here?

RACHEL. I think so.

NADIMA. Good. Good. And you? Do you…feel safe here?

RACHEL. Nadima? What are you asking me?

NADIMA. I spend my days...matching *souls* to homes. When you get down to it, that's what I do. Make the right fit between a spirit and a place where it can rest. *(Turns to* **RACHEL.***)* So?

RACHEL. Yes. I feel safe.

NADIMA. Good.

(*Beat.*)

Rachel...*my* soul? Doesn't match this home anymore.

RACHEL. Nadima...

NADIMA. Your family... Gut first, head second. I don't –

RACHEL. Yes. And *my* gut told me to be out there with that baby just now. Put an arm around her. Why weren't you?

(**NADIMA** *is speechless.*)

Your soul could fit if you wanted it to, Nadima.

NADIMA. *(Head in her hands.)* Don't know if that's true, baby.

RACHEL. Wow. *(Pause.)* Listen, you're gonna do what you wanna do. Kick us out, / run away,

NADIMA. *(Disbelief.)* I'm *not* kicking you out. / I wouldn't –

RACHEL. Stay out late. Drink with "clients" or whatever. I don't have that luxury. There's a little girl out there / that needs –

NADIMA. Rachel, you know, this whole time – from day ONE – I've made decisions that have pressed me further into her. That is a *true* thing, baby. *And* pressed me further into *you*. Because I love you. Changed the whole trajectory of my / life.

RACHEL. Whose life *hasn't* changed, Nadima?! *(Pause.)* You resented her the moment she walked through that door.

NADIMA. That's not –

RACHEL. Yes, it is. Walk around here with your face fixed in a frown all day. You think she can't see that? You think *I* can't?

NADIMA. How am I supposed to –? Rachel! *Every* time I extend my hand – I pack a lunch, I help with homework or –. EVERY TIME it's, "I got it, Nadima. I got it. That's not how you do it, Nadima. Let go. Let me." You slap my hand away!!!

RACHEL. Because help without joy can feel like a punishment, Nadima!

(Beat.)

Our job right now – regardless of all this mess – is to carve out *some* sense of joy for that kid as long as she's here. It's up to us to do that. *(Pause.)* Or is it up to me? Is it up me, Nadima?

NADIMA. I feel like you already made that decision, babe.

RACHEL. What?

NADIMA. *(Pause.)* It's like a tornado. And you all are spinning around in it like this is how it's *supposed* to be. And I just... But, you know my heart tells me, "Maybe you can stop some of the spinning if you just love this woman more. With everything you've got, Nadima. If you choose her. Over and over again. Even when she doesn't choose...[you]." Baby, I don't have the um –. And you push me away. 'Cause I don't *do* how you all do. This spinning. When it comes to your sister. To each other... You push me away. And I get it, Love.

RACHEL. Ain't nobody pushing you nowhere, Nadima!

NADIMA. You lock me out of my own bedroom, Rachel! Lock me out of the *bed* that I haven't been welcomed into for god knows how long, honey.

RACHEL. Don't you dare. You see what that baby is going through?!

NADIMA. I DO, RACHEL! I do, but you…you hold on to that little girl so tight. Like you're trying to *strangle* your sister's love and forgiveness out of her. *Squeeze* whatever mistakes you think you made, out of existence, from that tiny little body of hers. You are wrapped around her so firmly that there's no *room* for anything else. Not even how I love you. How *can* my soul fit? It can't…

RACHEL. Nadima –

NADIMA. I can't do what your family does, baby!

RACHEL. I'm not asking you to!

NADIMA. Aren't you?

(**RACHEL** *concedes.*)

RACHEL. *(Pitifully.)* What if *you* are my family?

NADIMA. *(Nods in acknowledgment.) And* I know what's supposed to happen. A kid comes along and all these maternal…juices are supposed to start flowing, but… And I tried. SO hard. It's not gonna be enough I think. Joy…

(*Beat.*)

I tried to. I really did. And, if I wasn't exactly a cheerful giver… I'm sorry about that. I am.

(*Beat.*)

But. *You* feel safe. And *Sam* feels safe. *(Fighting back tears.)* And that makes me *so* happy. *(Smiles.)* At least I had an instinct for *that*. To match your souls to someplace safe. At least you let me have that.

(**RACHEL** *weeps.*)

RACHEL. My Heart, I –

> (**NADIMA** *places her hand on* **RACHEL***'s heart. Wipes the tears from her eyes. Then, kisses her forehead.*)

NADIMA. Shh. Hey. He's gonna find her.

> (**NADIMA** *smiles reassuringly. Then kisses* **RACHEL** *longingly. Their foreheads meet for a held moment. She exits the apartment. Leaving* **RACHEL** *with the weight of this break.* **NADIMA** *catches* **SAM** *sitting alone on the stoop, deep in thought.* **NADIMA** *looks at her lovingly.* **SAM** *catches her eyes.* **NADIMA** *sits next to her. And they hold there in stillness. All three* **WOMEN** *are left in soft light and the heft of their thoughts. As the sound of a distant train is heard.*)

Scene Four

*(As the **WOMEN** hold, there is a break in the darkness. **REGGIE** sits on the crate just as we saw him at the end of the prologue. One of those vacant "behind the tracks" places, where Amtrak trains and Greyhound buses might store overnight, appears around him. A recent past. After a moment, **MONIQUE** enters as before. Hands in pockets and cool. She's seen better days. The sight of one another conjures up that familiar rhythm of when they were younger...)*

MONIQUE. Man, is you lookin' fah somebody?

REGGIE. *(Looks up to see his wife. A moment.)* You ain't gonna push me away?

MONIQUE. Ain't gonna push you.

REGGIE. *(Lovingly. Hesitantly.)* I'm gonna touch you. See if ya real.

MONIQUE. Come on then.

(He embraces her slowly. Then kisses her passionately. Deeply.)

REGGIE. You don't mind that?

MONIQUE. *(She melts.)* I don't mind.

*(Lights slowly fade on **RACHEL**, **NADIMA**, and **SAM**. They exit. **MONIQUE** carefully pulls away from **REGGIE**. Looks up at the sky. She pulls that familiar wrapped package **REGGIE** gave **SAM** from her jacket pocket. Hands it to **REGGIE**.)*

I signed yo name to it too. So it come from both 'a us.

(He takes it. Studies it.)

This ain't like home is it?

REGGIE. Ain't nothing like Vixten. *(Beat. Still examining the package.)* Had me out here lookin' fah ya. All these months. Like some damn fool, Monique.

(**MONIQUE** *studies her feet. Hands in pockets.*)

Your sistah call me, 'n I called them folks over in Tennessee. Ain't nobody seen ya. But, *you* don't call me til now…? That don't make no sense tah me, baby.

MONIQUE. *(A moment. Trying desperately to recapture a bit of past magic.)* Hm. Where you been? What you *seen*, Reggie?

REGGIE. What? Mean out looking for *you*?

MONIQUE. Yeah! What ya *seen*, man?

REGGIE. Neekie…

MONIQUE. Come on, Reggie. What you –?

REGGIE. *(Snaps.)* I don't know! Worst 'a the world sometimes cooped up in a men's shelter fah a night. Best of it in a hotel room offa 95. Bus stops. Smell 'a gasoline.

MONIQUE. *(Almost blissful.)* Yeah. Smell 'a gasoline. Colors. Music. Sound. When I was ridin' up to New York wit' Sam I had nothin' but a panic in my chest, ya know. Decided to go on over tah Tennessee first and see what the set up was. This *really* nice neighborhood just outside the city. Peaceful. But I looked at it and that panic got deeper… And I *knew* –

REGGIE. Knew you was gonna run away from me? Leave our baby? / That's what ya knew?

MONIQUE. I knew it wouldn't *work*, Reggie! They wanted to keep me cooped up in that big ole house. Day in. Day out. Track my every step. Tell me how *good* I was for tryin'. How *smart* 'n *important* 'n *special* 'n… Reggie… I already had that. With you. And that didn't work either.

REGGIE. You mockin' how I loved you?

MONIQUE. No, Reggie, no!

REGGIE. *(Unraveling a bit.)* We had a plan!

MONIQUE. *You* did. *You* had the plan, man! You always do!

REGGIE. Well, what the hell was yours?! You left me stranded wit' blood on my hands 'n you wanna stay lost?! I *don't* understand that, Neekie!

MONIQUE. You know it ain't had nothin' to do with the blood on your hands, Reggie. It's got everything to do with the blood on *hers*.

REGGIE. One and the same.

MONIQUE. No. No it ain't, baby. My lil girl standin' there wit' her father by her side. Her father who she *adores*. Wearin' the pain I caused *him* all over *her* face. Man who she would do anythang fah. / Am I right, Reggie?

REGGIE. She did that fah you!

MONIQUE. You taught her how to clean it. You taught her how to load it. And you taught her tah aim straight. Jus' like her Pa.

(Beat.)

REGGIE. You know it was s'posed tah be me who done it. Had it sittin' 'nere fah me on the table. Ready fah 'im. She picked it up 'fore I knew it.

MONIQUE. I know, Reggie. I know. And now what you gonna do? Cover it up *and* take her on the road wicha? Make her live with a strung-out woman she ain't never learn tah love noway? What, you gonna try and change that memory for her? Make it all go away? What's ya plan?

REGGIE. Look here... Maybe you come on up to your sister's with me? This ain't too far out. We'll tell them –

MONIQUE. Oh, Reggie… You just as bad as me. And what's worse you don't even know it.

REGGIE. What?

MONIQUE. What are you chasin' when you come huntin' after me? Look at you. You bad as me.

REGGIE. How you *talk* to me?

MONIQUE. I ain't nobody mama, Reggie…

REGGIE. *(Refuses to listen.)* We ain't but 'bout a hundred miles out! You can't live like this forever, / Neekie.

MONIQUE. Reggie. God…you bad as me.

REGGIE. If we just / TALK tah 'em –

MONIQUE. Stop it, Reggie / Stop.

REGGIE. You get yourself together –

MONIQUE. STOP! *(Pause.)* I done *tried*, Reggie! For years, I tried.

REGGIE. You ain't tried shit! You ran away! From *everything*! YOU! Shit! Every goddamn thing I stood up for or fought hard to build, you STAY *STEADY* TEARING that shit down!! / I ain't like you!

MONIQUE. I FUCKED IT UP! IT'S ON ME!! I FUCKED IT UP! I know that!! You right! You right, Reggie. I *been* tearing shit down from jump! It's what I knew to do, man. I HAD to run, Reggie. To put it back *together* somehow! What I got to give a child when all I know is what my mama give me? What I got to give *you*? Don't tell me I ain't tried! I brought that baby to meet her grandmama. Reached out to my mother with a dust of hope in my heart that she'd look at her grandbaby different than she did me. And I left my mother's house heart broke when she couldn't even find it in herself to glance over at her. I was broken even when you first come to me, Reggie. From my ROOT! You got to tend to the root. And it rotted, Reggie. ROTTED! When I left my mama house that last time I knew right then an' 'nere that...*my* lil girl was bound tah rot away too. 'Cause of me! 'Cause that what my mama give *me*. That ain't no home. Not with a mama dyin' on the inside of it like that.

REGGIE. God...dammit!! Who say you got tah be her? Who say ya couldna held ya daughter close 'n do the same for me?

> (**MONIQUE** *is short for words.*)

[You wanna know] what *I'm chasin'*? I ain't NONE 'a the thangs my daddy was 'cept HERE! That root was piss sour and mean as hell! I looked that man square in his eye when I was a boy 'n tole him tah his *face* I ain't never wanted tah be nothin' like 'im. I took all that Devil he put in me, wrapped him up 'n kicked its ass down the road. Like I shook that man's DNA outta me. The face of my father with no trace of him on the inside. I snip MY root clean off! That's me. What *I'm* chasin'. Who say you couldna done the same damn thang?

MONIQUE. (*Softly. With doubt.*) Ain't nobody say.

Ain't nobody.

> (*They sit for a bit knowing they are no longer one.* **REGGIE** *picks up the package. Studies it again. Looks at his wife.* **SAM** *enters from the bedroom.*)

Scene Five

*(Brooklyn. Lights rise on **SAM** who sits on the couch. Something has changed about her. Something is a little harder. Worn. **MONIQUE** and **REGGIE** are manifestations of her contemplation. A moment passes. As **MONIQUE** and **REGGIE** exit **RACHEL** enters from the bedroom and lingers in the doorway watching her niece. Finally...)*

RACHEL. Got any advice for a restless sleeper?

*(**SAM** doesn't answer.)*

God. I wish I could just lift some of that weight off of your shoulders, Sam. I so wish I could.

SAM. Weight must be good for somethin'.

RACHEL. You don't deserve it.

SAM. It's mine though. The more that's on me the deeper my feet sink into the ground. I guess.

RACHEL. I suppose so.

*(**RACHEL** spots the gift that **REGGIE** brought still sitting on the table.)*

Your daddy wrapped your gift real nice.

SAM. Yeah.

RACHEL. It's a little worn. Travelin' with him for so long. You wanna open it?

SAM. No. You can if you wanna.

*(**RACHEL** picks up the package and sits next to **SAM** on the couch.)*

RACHEL. Let's open it together.

SAM. What have I done, Aunt Rachel?

RACHEL. Sweetheart, you didn't do anything.

> *(Beat.)*

SAM. My parents. They like…a shadow to me.

RACHEL. How do you mean?

SAM. I can see 'em. I can see 'em but… I kinda *can't* really? It's on purpose I think. They act like they brung a child into the world with no eyes.

RACHEL. Well, what do you see?

SAM. *(Considers.)* They hurt.

RACHEL. Yes.

SAM. They scared?

And it's me. I done somethin'.

They scared 'a me.

RACHEL. No baby, they ain't scared of you. Sam, your mother was fourteen when she had you. Your father was fifteen. And I know that seems like a very long time away from how old you are now but that isn't old. Me? Now, that's old. Believe me, honey they took everything they knew and learned in that little bit of years about love and family and the world and they poured as much of that as they could into you. Sometimes it's sweet like candy. Or a bit…unfair. Sometimes it is really unfair the things that get poured into you. And *their* unfair started taking over their sweet. *That's* what scares them. What they had left in them to pour. Not you. But, look here. You are here with me now and I am not perfect. I cannot promise you perfection but I would love it if you would allow me to continue to pour every ounce of love that I can into you? I would really really appreciate that Sam.

(SAM softens, but barely looks at RACHEL.)

There's a card. Why don't you read it to me?

(She gives the card to SAM.)

SAM. "A lil somethin' from ya Ma and Dad." *(She opens it.)* It's all crinkly.

RACHEL. Been in his bag more than a minute I s'pose.

SAM. *(She reads.)* "Fah when ya mouth can't find the words tah let ya feelings show...

Keep this near you.

Add to it.

And we will never be apart.

We love you, baby girl. Breathe."

RACHEL. Pretty paper. Why don't you pull this end here?

(SAM pulls the ribbon from the package.)

There you go. And I'll peel this back. Oh.

(They open it to reveal a worn notebook. RACHEL starts to tear up.)

SAM. What's wrong?

RACHEL. Nothing. Nothing it's... this, Samantha McCloud Barber... this is Monique McCloud's journal. Her notebook. She wrote in it every day. Starting from when she was a few years younger than you are right now.

SAM. My mom?

RACHEL. My sister. Your mother. Yes. Your mother is the most beautiful writer. Did you know that?

(SAM shrugs.)

RACHEL. She wrote all of the time. On anything she could get her hands on and your grandmother got so tired of finding bits of paper and napkins all over her house and finally brought home this journal for her. "Keep it all in one place and offa my floor!" she said. Look at this. See here?

SAM. Look how tiny her handwriting is.

RACHEL. She didn't want to waste space.

(She flips through the pages.)

Let's find something... oh it's marked here. What's that say?

*(She hands over the book to **SAM**.)*

SAM. "Awaiting."

RACHEL. Can you read it?

SAM.
This is Dawnin'
All hands assume the position
In praise 'a her comin'.
Peasants' knees bent in welcome.
An obedient *(Sounding out the word.)* Per – cher – on

*(**MONIQUE** appears in Vixten, Georgia. Fourteen. Pregnant. Beautiful.)*

What's a Percheron?

RACHEL. It's a kind of horse. Very strong. Very beautiful.

SAM & MONIQUE.
An obedient Percheron nudges tha Lion
Tah bow his head in homage.

MONIQUE. *(Continues to recite the piece. Addressing her belly.)*

Knights' and Warriors' supinated grips hold steady

Tha varied lengths 'a tha Horizon's edge as

We

Wait

Fah Her.

A Willow tree branch's unexpected reach

Upward

Tickles tha air 'n purifies a now jubilant Win'[d]

So She

May breathe

Joy.

Tha Earth checks its pace.

Tha Moon winks tah test the twinkle 'a her servant Stars.

And Nāycha [Nature]

Sets a table

Full 'a bounty

So She

May go no days wantin'.

And we wait

Patiently.

No need for anxious coaxin'.

She knows how tah make a' entrance.

The grandest 'a ladies do.

She has granted Grace tha honor

'a serving Her as escort.

Tha decision is Hers

In fact

MONIQUE & RACHEL.
In fact

> (*The lights fade on* **MONIQUE**. *As* **RACHEL** *reads.*)

RACHEL.
No *Mother* chooses a chil'

For when Grace is given his command

He acts as carrier

Sending notice of a calling

To the Mother,

That final hue in a symphony of verdant readiness,

Who obeys

And waits

For Her

> (**SAM** *is overcome. She flips through the pages. Trying to find her mother in them. A different kind of anger.*)

SAM. How come…? How come…? Where is she, Aunt Rach? I can't… (*Exhales. Cries.*) Where is she?

> (**SAM** *falls into her* **AUNT**. *She breaks into tears.*)

Scene Six

(A new day. That same vacant "behind the tracks" place. **REGGIE** *and* **MONIQUE** *stare into the night air.)*

MONIQUE. Moon happy tonight. Lit up almost like daytime.

REGGIE. Hmph.

(Beat.)

MONIQUE. You give it to her? She open it?

REGGIE. *(Smiles painfully.)* I left it d'ere wit' her yeah. Still wrapped pretty sittin' on the table when I left.

MONIQUE. *(Closes her eyes.)* Man… I remember the… pencil in my hand. Pages 'a mine 'n pages 'a somebody else's. But those words…? I lost her.

REGGIE. Sam'll find her.

MONIQUE. You think so?

(He nods yes.)

Good. That's…good.

That's the girl ya fell in love wit' ain't it?

REGGIE. Yes.

MONIQUE. *(As much for herself as it is for* **SAM.***)* Yeah. I hope she find her.

(Beat.)

Thank you, Reggie. I jus' wanted tah see ya again. I'm glad I did. Where are / you – [headed]?

REGGIE. *(Stern. Cold.)* What you gonna do?

MONIQUE. I made me a picture list 'a all the places –

REGGIE. *(Sharply.)* 'Cause it seem tah me ya gotta coupla choices. Head on back up tah Tennessee 'n spit on the Devil or settle in on bein' a sour root.

MONIQUE. *(A pained smile.)* I got me a plan.

REGGIE. Ain't mine tah make fah ya no more.

MONIQUE. *(Softly.)* I ain't asking ya to.

*(**MONIQUE** starts to head off.)*

REGGIE. Hol' up.

(He can't help it. He hands her some money. She refuses it.)

Come on nah.

MONIQUE. No –

REGGIE. I said, come on nah!

(She reluctantly takes it.)

I ain't gonna tell ya what tah do wit' it.

MONIQUE. Steady tryna fix thangs.

REGGIE. *(A heartbroken smile.)* Jus' let me get this last one in here... I got to keep it moving. Ain't no tellin' when somebody gonna come 'round askin' questions. Ya better go on too.

(Beat.)

I ain't throwin' you away.

MONIQUE. I know.

(They kiss.)

REGGIE. I ain't got it in me tah throw you away.

*(The soft sounds of rhythmic hand clapping and laughter start to fill the space. **MONIQUE** sets herself to leave.)*

MONIQUE. Did she seem happy?

REGGIE. I tol' you –

MONIQUE. My sister? Rachel. She look like she happy Sam 'nere?

> *(Lights slowly fade up on* **RACHEL** *and* **SAM** *playing "Sophisticated Lady.")*

REGGIE. I think we did right by our little girl. I do.

MONIQUE. Good.

> *(She walks away getting smaller and smaller in the distance.* **REGGIE** *lingers then walks in the opposite direction. Duffle bag over his shoulder. He fades away.)*
>
> *(A bright clear sunny day in Brooklyn appears. Out on the street. Sound of kids playing. Music and cars passing by.* **SAM** *and* **RACHEL** *in mid-laughter as they continue playing.)*

RACHEL & SAM.
Sophisticated lady

That's me

Sophisticated lady

That's me

Well my

SAM.
Name is Sammie

RACHEL & SAM.
And I'm

SAM.
Short and fine

RACHEL & SAM.
　If you

SAM.
　Tip me over

RACHEL & SAM.
　I will

SAM.
　Blow your mind

RACHEL & SAM.
　I got

SAM.
　Hips to party

RACHEL & SAM.
　And I

SAM.
　Love my man

RACHEL & SAM.
　If you

SAM.
　Try and take him

RACHEL & SAM.
　I'll do

SAM.
　All I can

RACHEL & SAM.
　I'll do

SAM.
　All I can

RACHEL & SAM.
　Sophisticated lady
　That's me

Sophisticated lady

That's me

RACHEL. Sophisticated hunh? Oh, you think you grown now?

SAM. *(Shyly. Resisting a smile.)* I don't know.

RACHEL. You *is* big now, Sam.

Let that smile out, girl!

I see it. Ohhh sookie sookie I see it!

> *(She can't help it.* **SAM** *breaks into a huge smile. It's a release she desperately needs.)*

There it is!

> *(***SAM***'s laughter is so rich and full, so alive that it seems to conjure the image that forms slowly in the background.* **RACHEL** *sees it. It's her sister in silhouette.* **RACHEL** *turns to her and is at once her teenage self.)*

(To **MONIQUE***.)* Hey, little girl.

MONIQUE. *(To* **SAM***.)* Hey, little girl.

> *(***SAM** *turns toward her mother's voice.)*

RACHEL. *(To* **MONIQUE***.)* I gotta be moving on. School.

MONIQUE. *(To* **RACHEL***.)* Dey got school *here!*

Can't you stay? Please?

SAM. *(To* **MONIQUE***.)* Can't you stay?

RACHEL. *(To* **MONIQUE***.)* You gonna be all right, little girl.

I know it.

MONIQUE. *(To* **SAM***.)* You gonna be all right.

I can't stay here, baby.

RACHEL. *(To* **MONIQUE***.)* I just want to tell you…

MONIQUE. *(To* **SAM.***)* I just want you to know...

I'm... I'm sorry

RACHEL. *(To* **MONIQUE.***)* I am so so sorry.

MONIQUE. *(To* **SAM.***)* And I love you, little girl.

RACHEL. *(To* **MONIQUE.***)* I love you, little sister.

You 'bout the smartest kid I know.

MONIQUE. *(To* **SAM.** *She starts to walk away.)* You are my baby girl.

SAM. *(To* **MONIQUE.** *Shyly.)* Wait! Please

I...want to teach you a game.

MONIQUE. *(To* **RACHEL.***)* I got a new game!

RACHEL. *(To* **MONIQUE.***)* Something mama taught you?

MONIQUE. *(To* **SAM.***)* Something your pa taught you?

SAM. *(Shyly. To* **MONIQUE.***)* Something I came up with myself.

MONIQUE. *(Smiles. To* **RACHEL.***)* Something I wrote.

RACHEL. *(To* **MONIQUE.***)* Sure, little sister.

MONIQUE. *(To* **SAM.***)* Sure, baby teach me.

*(***SAM** *gets her mother's journal from the stoop.)*

SAM. *(To* **MONIQUE** *and* **RACHEL.***)* It's real easy. Stand right here.

(The **WOMEN** *form a circle.* **SAM** *orchestrates the* **WOMEN** *from the instructions she has written in the journal.)*

Put one hand up and one hand down like this.

(She shows them.)

There you go. Good. Now, we're gonna tap each other's hands like this while we sing then clap on our own for two, okay?

MONIQUE. *(To **RACHEL**.)* I think I might actually know this one.

RACHEL. *(To **MONIQUE** and **SAM**.)* Oh, I know this game!

SAM. *(To **MONIQUE** and **RACHEL**. Places the journal down.)* You know the hand motions. I changed the words. Just repeat after me.

(Sings.)

Red clay, Red clay

RACHEL & MONIQUE.
Red clay, Red clay

SAM.
Under my feet

RACHEL & MONIQUE.
Under my feet

SAM.
Changed it all

RACHEL & MONIQUE.
Changed it all

SAM.
For a city street

RACHEL & MONIQUE.
For a city street

SAM.
Breathing hard

RACHEL & MONIQUE.
Breathing hard

SAM.
>Can't get no rest

RACHEL & MONIQUE.
>Can't get no rest

SAM.
>Got a ghost of time

RACHEL & MONIQUE.
>Got a ghost of time

SAM.
>Sittin' on my chest

RACHEL & MONIQUE.
>Sittin' on my chest

>>(**SAM** *slowly breaks away and plays this hand game by herself.* **RACHEL** *and* **MONIQUE** *stand in awe of* **SAM**.)

SAM.
>Maybe one day
>Someday soon

RACHEL & MONIQUE.
>Maybe one day
>Someday soon

SAM.
>I'll see my mama
>In the middle of the moon

RACHEL & MONIQUE.
>I'll see my mama
>In the middle of the moon

>>(*As* **SAM** *continues,* **MONIQUE** *slowly fades away into the background.* **RACHEL** *sits on her haunches gazing up at her niece. Lights fade on* **RACHEL**. **SAM** *alone.*)

SAM.
>Maybe one day
>Someday soon
>
>I'll see my mama
>In the middle of the moon
>
>Maybe one day
>Someday soon
>
>I'll see my mama
>In the middle of the moon
>
>Walk tall, little girl
>Jump up
>
>Walk tall, little girl
>Jump up
>
>Walk tall, little girl
>Jump up
>
>Walk tall, little girl
>Jump up

End of Play

www.ingramcontent.com/pod-product-compliance
Lightning Source LLC
Chambersburg PA
CBHW072014290426
44109CB00018B/2230